C000179061

LOSE A STONE IN JANUARY

THE ULTIMATE WEIGHT-LOSS AND WELLNESS PLAN

JACQUELINE WHITEHART

PEPIK BOOKS

Pepik Books

York

www.52recipes.co.uk

A catalogue record for this book is
available from the British Library.
ISBN: 978-0-9955318-4-0

This book features weight-loss techniques which may not
be suitable for everyone. You should always consult with a
qualified medical practitioner before starting any weight-loss
programme, or if you have any concerns about your health.
This book is not tailored to individual requirements or needs
and its contents are solely for general information purposes.
It should not be taken as professional or medical advice or
diagnosis. The activities detailed in this book should not be used
as a substitute for any treatment or medication prescribed or
recommended to you by a medical practitioner. The author and
the publishers do not accept any responsibility for any adverse
effects that may occur as a result of the use of the suggestions
or information herein. If you feel that you are experiencing
adverse effects after embarking on any weight-loss programme,
including the type described in this book, it is imperative that
you seek medical advice. Results may vary from individual to
individual.

LOSE A STONE IN JANUARY

Lose a Stone in January

LOSE A STONE IN JANUARY

The Ultimate Weight-loss and Wellness Plan

Do you feel sluggish and blue after the Christmas and new year excesses? Are you in need of a health reboot? Want the perfect plan for your dry January?

The January weight-loss and wellness plan gives you a diet plan tailored to improve your metabolism, a range of simple and delicious recipes that are easy to follow and suit all tastes and budgets and aN easy-to follow exercise plan that is suitable for all abilities.

- Real weight-loss that lasts
- Healthy and safe
- Helps blood sugar, cholesterol and energy
- Three balanced meals a day
- Clear advice that works
- Over 50 fresh and simple recipes

INTRODUCTION

A New Approach

This unique plan is designed to give you 3 proper meals a day so you won't go hungry.

Each day of the diet is nutritionally balanced so you are getting plenty of lean protein, good fats, smart carbs and a variety of fruit and vegetables. The plan is divided into different phases, each lasting four days. The phases are Detox and De-stress, Proteins & Healthy Fats, Better Carbs, Balanced Eating. It's important to note that this plan is about moderation not deprivation. So you'll still be eating some carbs during the Protein & Healthy Fats phase and vice versa. So get ready to join a new diet revolution (it's a revolution because you don't have to go hungry on this diet!), enjoy the delicious and healthy meal choices and let the results speak for themselves.

This diet is not about starving yourself, it's about sticking to a plan and working together to achieve the same goal.

That's right, I'll be working with you right through the plan. Most people (but not everyone) find it easier to work towards their goals with the help of others - that feeling of not being alone is very powerful.

With this in mind, I'll be introducing various tools to

motivate and encourage everyone taking part in this programme. These are all totally free to use and you can dip in and out as you want.

To sign up for regular motivational emails with tips, recipes and non-judgemental encouragement you just need to sign up here:

http://www.52recipes.co.uk/january

If you follow that link you'll also find info on how to join our Facebook group to meet and swap tips with your fellow dieters.

THE PLAN

Seven different phases, each four days long, makes one powerful month

This plan is all about shaking it up. Making you feel differently about what you eat and how you eat. Have you ever been told to mix up your exercise routine because your muscles 'get used to it'? It's the same with your diet, you need a burst of change every few days or your body gets used to it and you stop seeing results.

What do I mean by that? If you only ever do one form of exercise, like running or spinning, your body gets used to that exercise and you stop seeing results. You're using the same muscles every day and neglecting all the other muscles in your body. In the same way that a change of exercise routine keeps your body surprised and gets you over the hump, a change in your nutrition programme every few days shakes up your metabolism and keeps the weight-loss going.

This programme ensures that you never have more than 4 days eating in the same way. Your body keeps working, keeps breaking down fat and wakes up your sluggish metabolism.

Eat different = lose weight (It's as simple as that)

THE PLAN AT A GLANCE

Detox and de-stress (Days 1-4)

Proteins and healthy fats 1 (Days 5-8)

Better carbs 1 (Days 9-12)

Protein and healthy fats 2 (Days 13-16)

Better carbs 2 (Days 17-20)

Protein and healthy fats 3 (Days 21-24)

Balanced eating for your metabolism (Days 25-28)

Different phases help you shift fat faster

Let's consider how the four phases of the Weight-loss and Wellness programme coax your body to burn fat, build muscle and lay the foundation for a healthier you.

Our bodies require variety in the foods we eat in order to function correctly. You need carbohydrates, natural sugars, protein, fat and salt to maintain normal body chemistry. At times you'll need higher therapeutic levels of these elements, especially when you've been depriving yourself for too long. Including these fuels, but not all at the same time, helps you to rebuild, restore and replenish your body. You will eat more, eat better and lose weight.

What about calories in, calories out?

I know some of my readers are going to complain that the recipes are not calorie counted. It happens time and time again. 'Please can I have the calories for 'myfitnesspal?' Or 'I need the calories so that I make sure I eat less than 1500 calories a day.'

I could count the calories in every recipe in the book. I have in the past calorie counted all recipes and ingredients. I will try and explain here why it's really important to NOT count calories, as it's counter-productive to all our weight-loss goals.

The number of calories is perhaps the least nutritionally interesting thing on the label. By weight, carbohydrates have the least calories, then protein and lastly fat. So by taking just calories as our guide we are restricting the filling proteins and fats and eating more sweet and starchy carbs. The problem: carbs don't fill you up. You need to eat more of them and the tendency to snack between meals is much increased.

I simply don't believe in the 'calories in < calories out = weight-loss' equation any more. You might think I'm crazy and you might even be cross with me for saying it but it's true.

A calorie is not a little ball or smartie that you pop into your mouth and when you've had 2000 or 2500 smarties you have had your quota for the day. This is a gross over-simplification and simply doesn't ring true in the real world. A calorie is just energy or the potential to provide energy.

In the real world, a calorie is not a set thing. Every person has a unique biochemical make up - so a calorie isn't going to be the same thing for you as it is for anyone else. What really matters, much more than the number of theoretical 'calories' you do or don't consume, is how you burn the food or otherwise distribute the energy, once it gets inside you.

A banana versus a low-calorie snack bar

If you just count calories you could well find that the snack bar has less calories than the banana and reach the conclusion that it is better for your diet. Wrong! The snack bar just has empty sweet carbohydrate calories. You'd be missing out on the dietary fibre, potassium, manganese and vitamin B6 that are packed into the banana.

A low-fat fruit yogurt vs a full fat natural yogurt

If you look at just the calorie information on these yogurts you'll find that the natural yogurt almost always comes up higher on the calories. Why? Because natural yogurt has more fat than the processed version and as we all know, fat is calorie dense. So in the manufacturing of a flavoured yogurt, the fat is stripped out and replaced with sweeteners, flavourings and thickeners. A fruit yogurt might have 10 or more ingredients while a natural one - only one.

With a few exceptions, the ingredients you use will either be fresh with no packaging eg. Fresh fruit and veg, meat from the butcher; or packaged one ingredient items, for example, a tin of tomatoes, a packet of oats or a pot of natural yogurt. If a packaged item contains more than three ingredients then it probably shouldn't have a place in your diet, either now on the programme or into the future.

Three Meals a Day, No Snacks

This is perhaps the most important tenet of the weight-loss plan.

There's plenty of meal choices for each phase of the diet - at least 5 choices for breakfast, lunch and dinner. You'll find simple options for one, couple-friendly meals for two and bigger meals consisting of 4 portions or more, which are suitable for keeping or freezing in batches. There's always a few vegetarian options and in an emergency you should check out the *Tips & Cheat Meals* section for each phase.

Every breakfast, lunch and dinner is designed to fill you up and keep you full until the next meal. The crux of the matter is that you simply won't feel hungry between meals so it's easy to not snack.

If you DO fancy a snack, ask yourself are you really hungry? Many of us reach for whatever treats we can find during the 'danger times' of mid-afternoon and late evening and this is one of the most common causes of slow but steady weight-gain. The most important thing we can do is break this habit over the diet programme. It will get us a long way towards achieving our weight-loss goal and enable us to maintain the weight-loss when the programme is over.

Guidelines for each phase

The basic tenets of the different phases are the same:

1   Eat 3 meals a day
2   Don't snack between meals
3   Follow the recipes for each stage
4   No alcohol
5   Each phase lasts 4 days

As well as the balance of the meals you eat there are also some 'do's and don'ts' for each phase.

Detox and De-stress: Guidelines

The balance we are hoping for in this phase is

Carbs: 50 / Protein: 30 / Fats: 20

Your overall food consumption will go down during this phase to allow your body to recover from any excesses. Don't worry: daily consumption goes up as soon as you reach the next phase.

A little bit of fruit as part of or after each and every meal is encouraged. Allowed fruits are apples, grapefruit, oranges, satsumas, strawberries (4), raspberries (10), blackberries (10), blueberries (25) and kiwi. In fact most fresh fruit is allowed, with the exception of banana as this contains more sugar and starch than other fruits.

Avoid all sugar that is not naturally occuring.

Also steer clear of red meats in all forms and keep fatty foods such as cheese in moderation.

No chocolate...not even dark...yet.

If you're a caffeine addict this is when you'll be decompressing from your caffeine addiction as you move towards minimal caffeine in the form of green or white tea. If you haven't managed to cut back before you start then do it gradually during this first phase. Drink one cup less per day until you reach your goal.

Protein & Healthy Fats: Guidelines

The balance we are hoping for in this phase is

Carbs: 20 / Protein: 40 / Fats: 40

If you have a sweet tooth then this is probably the phase you'll find most challenging. This is because anything that is sweet, including naturally sweet fruit and yogurt, contains more carbs than we would like during the Protein and Healthy Fats phase. Vegetables are not restricted, even though they contain some carbohydrate and salad fruits (I'm talking tomatoes) are also allowed.

If you want to include one portion of fruit - think berries or citrus - into your breakfast routine then this is encouraged. But fruit later in the day, even with meals, should be avoided. The same can be said of natural yogurt or (better) quark, a small portion can be incorporated into breakfast but not later in the day.

Again avoid all sweet foods including chocolate.

Better Carbs: Guidelines

The balance we are hoping for during this phase is

Carbs: 40 / Protein: 40 / Fats: 20

The better carbs phase is the most relaxed phase when it comes to satisfying your sweet tooth. Don't get too excited, as it is necessary to continue to steer clear of the obvious cakes and biscuits. But fruit in moderation - up to 3 portions a day - preferably with meals but could be allowed as a mid-afternoon pick me up.

And also... here comes chocolate. The dark (70%) kind is definitely allowed. That's 6 squares (20g) per day. After meals is best but how you split it is up to you. Just make sure you enjoy every mouthful really slowly. Take a small bit, pop it in your mouth and allow to melt on your tongue.

Balanced Eating: Guidelines

Don't feel confused by the Balanced Eating phase. It is a transitional phase from a strict programme to carrying on good practice after the diet. You should follow the basic tenets for the programme: 3 meals a day, no snacks, no alcohol. But you can pick any recipe from each of the previous phases. Pick your favourites, try something new, whatever you fancy. The 'Tips and Cheat Meals' from each phase are also open to you.

THE PHASES IN DETAIL

Detox and De-stress: What to expect?

Detox and De-stress is the first phase of the programme, lasting for 4 days. The aim is to cut out toxic foods and allow our bodies to prepare for the important fat-burning stages to come.

This first phase is perhaps the one that we most recognise as 'diety' as the foods are lighter than during other phases. The foods provide you with enough energy to get you through the day but perhaps not much to spare. If you've been used to eating a lot over the Christmas period you might think 'Is this it?' with the smaller portions and junk-free food. This first phase is a bit of a wake up call. How much weight have you put on over Christmas - 7 pounds, a stone, more...? You have to break those habits and do it now or else the weight will still be there for the summer or even ready for next Christmas.

There are a lot of positives too. Some of that extra fat will just fall off as soon as you start to detox. Your body knows it has a few extra reserves and uses them up first. Your motivation will be high and you should lose a couple of pounds just in the first few days. That's a great way to start your diet and set yourself up for your target of a stone within the darkest month of January.

What to expect in the Detox & De-stress phase?

Will I be hungry? Possibly yes a bit during danger times like the evenings. It's not real hunger though, just habit. Break it now!

Other possible side effects of the Detox & De-stress Phase

- Headaches from caffeine withdrawal.

If you've been drinking a lot of caffeine and you cut down to next to nothing then it is likely you'll get a caffeine withdrawal headache during the first few days of the diet. Help to mitigate this by either cutting down before during the preparation days or cut back one cup at a time. So if Day One is 6 cups of tea, Day Two is 5 cups etc. It is obviously best to start cutting back as soon as you can, preferably during the preparation stage.

- A few more spots.

This really isn't the diet programme's fault, it's all the rich Christmas food. When you cut out the bad fats and sugars, your body starts its own detox programme and that can include spots. It will be over by the end of week one and when they've passed your skin will look healthier and more radiant - I promise!

And the positives...

- Noticeable weight-loss in just 4 days
- Better sleep

With no booze, caffeine or heavy food you'll sleep

better and look healthier straight away. It will lift your mood and make dieting so much easier too.

• Shaking it up.

It's just 4 days and then you move onto a more calorific (but better for fat-burning) phase in *Proteins and Healthy Fats*.

Proteins and Healthy Fats

Proteins and Healthy Fats is perhaps the most important phase of the "Lose a Stone Programme". It occurs three times during the plan, but never in succession. The phases are Phase 2: Days 5-8, Phase 4: Days 13-16, Phase 6: 21-24.

The fallacy I want to put to bed straight away is that just because this is the Protein and Fats phase, it doesn't mean that there will be no carbohydrate. Cutting out carbs entirely would mean cutting out fruit and veg and lovely things like yogurts and lentils. So instead think of this as the reduced carb phase. The difference here is that there are no 'just carbs' here, in either their starchy or sweet form. So while in other phases of the plan, there may be rice or potatoes for example, there'll be no ingredients that are almost exclusively carbs. However, you will find that smaller amounts of carbohydrates are allowed.

As a general rule, the food you eat in this phase will be roughly balanced in the ratio:

40% protein, 40% fat and 20% carb

What to expect during the Proteins and Healthy Fats phase?

During this phase you'll have very little sugar, only the natural sugar found in some fruit and yogurt. So if you are a sweet food junkie you might find this harder and you might get some cravings, especially in the evenings.

However, you'll also notice that you are not particularly hungry between meals so treat the cravings as what they are - a challenge to be overcome - rather than a real need.

Some of you diet junkies will find it really hard to up your protein and fat intake - you'll feel its going against years of 'dieting'. Ask yourself why you want to take part in this diet, why you still feel the need to lose weight after many years of dieting. Remember this plan is about shaking it up and breaking with tradition to find a healthier path to weight-loss.

Yes you'll feel fuller and more satisfied after meals, but that doesn't mean that you'll put on weight. By actually satiating yourself with a full balanced meal, your body relaxes, it's not in starvation mode anymore. So the overall effect is reduced hunger and suddenly your success rate shoots up and you can carry the programme through to the end. It's such a simple concept but be warned it can mess with your head if you've had years of 'diet programming'.

Because our society is so carbohydrate driven, you will find it harder to buy foods when you are out and about that are friendly to the Proteins and Healthy Fats phase. I was in Costa the other day and there was literally nothing suitable for me to eat. For that reason, you should plan more carefully for the Proteins and Healthy Fats phase. Take a good look at the recipes and choose a few that you think you'll really love. Look for ones that make several portions then you can have leftovers the next day rather than doing lots and lots of cooking.

Bizarrely the meal that is often the hardest during the proteins and healthy fats phase is breakfast. This is because breakfast is often a very carbohydrate based meal so swapping to high protein is harder. Chicken for breakfast? Not on my watch! First of all I would highly recommend eggs for breakfast or lunch during this phase (but not both!) A simple omelette is a really satisfying breakfast and can be ready in as long as it takes to make a slice of toast. So if you're stuck go for the omelette option for breakfast. I've also made sure the Tips and Cheats meals is really full of simple ideas for food choices during this phase because if you're not fully prepared this phase will be the hardest to follow when you're out and about.

I know many of you know how to cook the perfect omelette but for any of you that need a few pointers here's exactly how I do it at home:

Heat a generous drizzle (about a teaspoon) of olive oil in a heavy-based frying pan for a minute or two, before adding well-beaten eggs. Let the eggs cook a little before using a plastic spatula to pick up the sides of the omelette and letting the still runny centre go towards the edges. When just cooked (still a little wobbly in the middle), season with salt and pepper and fold in half before tipping onto a plate. It's ready in 2 minutes at and I usually just wipe round the pan with some kitchen paper rather than washing it with soapy water; this will mean it's well-oiled for the next day.

Better Carbs

Better Carbs occurs twice in the programme: Phase 3 (Days 9-12) and Phase 5 (Days 17-20).

Better Carbs is also perhaps a little different from what you expect. It's not about reducing fat and increasing carbs. Yes the balance tips towards carbs again, with approximately 40% of your daily nutrition intake coming from carbs. But there is still a significant proportion coming from protein (40%) and fats (20%).

Instead the focus of this stage is on the quality of the carbs consumed. As in the rest of the programme, carbs from wheat and sugar are cut back to the minimum amount. What we increase is the good carbs. Here's a list of my Top 10 Good Carbs. Never fear, the recipe section for this phase is absolutely choc full of good carbs so no need to worry about it too much - just get stuck into the delicious recipes.

The Good Carb List

Rice

Brown rice and basmati rice are both good carbohydrates. Brown rice has more fibre so is slightly better than basmati. If you find that the cooking time for brown rice is off-putting, try buying the pouches of pre-steamed rice that go from packet to plate in 2 minutes at. I like Tilda Brown Basmati rice as it has no unexpected ingredients.

Oats

Oats contain a very special and unique ingredient: beta-glucan. Beta-glucan is a type of fibre that means our bodies digest the carbohydrate more slowly and evenly. Oats therefore release their energy more slowly than other carbs and keep us fuller for longer. Oats are particularly good as a breakfast ingredient as they are so filling. Porridge oats are the standard oats we buy for porridge. Be careful to avoid 'quick' or 'express' oats as these have been overly processed with a lot of the goodness removed. Jumbo oats are bigger than porridge oats and have an even lower sugar load. They are also known as whole, traditional or old-fashioned oats.

Oat bran is the most concentrated form of beta-glucan. It's finely milled and is a great baking ingredient.

Potatoes

Choosing the right sort of potatoes is crucial. New potatoes boiled in their skins and a potato baked in its skin are good carbs. Mashed potato and chips are bad carbs. They key is in the skin, which adds fibre, texture and flavour. A good portion size is 150g – 3–4 new potatoes or a small jacket potato. This means that the all-time winter warmer of jacket potato, baked beans and cheese is a good option – just don't forget to eat the potato skin.

Butternut Squash

Butternut squash has a much lower impact on blood sugar than similar foods such as sweet potato and pumpkin. It's tasty and naturally sweet and goes really well in a range of vegetarian dishes or as a side dish with meat or fish.

Lentils

Lentils are an amazing blend of good carbohydrate and protein. They are also extremely versatile. Puy lentils are great in all kinds of stews and salads, adding a unique nutty flavour and texture. Red and brown lentils are used in a lot of Indian cooking. They make a great main vegetarian dish.

Quinoa

Quinoa is another food that mixes carbohydrate and protein. A simple grain without much taste of its own, use it as a meal accompaniment or anywhere you might previously have used couscous.

Chickpeas

Chickpeas are the most versatile and well balanced of the foods that mix carbs, fibre and protein. Use them to make falafel or in stews.

Beans

Kidney beans, cannellini beans – even baked beans – they're all good. If you're buying baked beans, check the ingredients list for too many nasties – look for varieties with reduced sugar and salt.

Nuts of all types

Nuts contain varying amounts of carbohydrates and usually quite a lot of good fat. They are very filing and do not raise your blood sugar by any signicant amount. They therefore make a great snack.

Dark Chocolate

Saving the best until last! Dark chocolate (70% cocoa solids) is a really good carbohydrate. It contains some sugary carbs but this is diluted by a good proportion of fibre. Use in cooking or snack on a few squares when you feel a craving.

Balanced Eating

Think of the last phase, Balanced Eating, as a stepping stone from the programme to the big wide world of healthy eating. Use all the tips and recipes you have learned in the earlier stages of the programme and put them together in a way that suits you. All recipes and eating choices from previous phases apply. For example, you can eat a meal from the Proteins and Healthy Fats phase and follow that with fruit or chocolate. Stick to the overall tenets of the programme - good carbs, 3 balanced meals a day, no alcohol.

The hope is that when you reach the end of the month, you'll be able to carry on some or all of the practices you have learnt. If you continue to incorporate some of the recipes into your diet, and keep snacks to a minimum then you will easily maintain the weight-loss you have achieved.

Towards the end of the phase and the diet, then it's time to have a look at yourself and see what you have achieved. If you weighed yourself at the start of the programme, then Day 28 (or perhaps the day after) is the time to get back on the scales and see how much weight you have lost. Of course this will vary person-to-person, some will have lost over a stone, some less, but every single person who has followed the programme will have lost weight, including shifting some of that stubborn belly fat.

Other changes that you might notice are:

- A more radiant, clear complexion
- Longer, deeper sleep
- Better mood
- Reduced anxiety and stress

GETTING STARTED

31 days in January

January has 31 days. We all know this. It tends to drag doesn't it? This plan is only 28 days long. There's a very good reason for that. We enter January with a bump and probably a hang over from the night before. It is not a good day to start a weight-loss program. To make it much much easier to follow I would recommend starting the programme on January 4th (that's a Wednesday in 2017). There's plenty to be getting on with in those first 3 days. Giving up alcohol and getting plenty of rest should be top of the list.

If you want to make a success of this amazing weight-loss programme then a gentle detox over the first 3 days of the year will make the programme so much easier. It's like running down a hill instead of jumping off a cliff!

Preparation

A week before you start you need to think about three things: buying a few specialist ingredients (either online or from a health food shop), cutting back your caffeine intake, and reducing your alcohol consumption.

If you look at the recipes, the vast majority of ingredients are readily available from the supermarket or local shops. Have a look for green and white tea - you'll be amazed how many different tea options are available now. White tea is like green tea but with a milder taste - definitely worth a look as it has all the some healthy essences. Also see if there are any fruit flavours that you fancy. You might just find your perfect beverage!

There is one recipe on the list that I heartily recommend and that is Chia Choc Granola - it's so healthy and filling and suitable for all phases except Protein and Healthy Fats. The granola requires two ingredients that may not be available at your local supermarket: chia seeds and malt extract. The first is chia seeds. These are tiny, virtually tasteless black seeds, similar to poppy seeds in appearance. Chia seeds are rich in protein and fibre and make a noticeable difference to your hunger levels after breakfast. They help the granola keep you full until lunchtime and beyond. (My local Sainsbury's has just started stocking chia so maybe your supermarket will too.)

The second ingredient is malt extract. If you are of a certain age, you may remember this as something you were fed by the spoonful as a small child. Malt extract is used in various recipes including the granola. Malt extract is a natural maltose sweetener. It is less 'sweet' than sugar but doesn't give you the sweet highs and lows of normal sugar. As a bonus it has a rich malty taste that really adds flavour to your cooking. Both chia seeds and malt extract can be found at any good health food shop in the UK and are relatively inexpensive. I purchased both from Holland & Barrett which has outlets in most towns and cities and has a great online shop too.

If you are not located in the UK, then these may also be the ingredients you struggle to find. Please get in touch as soon as you can if there are ingredients that are not easily accessible for you. Suitable alternatives can definitely be found but they will vary country by country. By letting me know what's difficult for you, I can help you source the right foods for you and also help me assist others in the future.

The next thing to think about in the week before you start the "Lose A Stone in January" programme is to cut back your caffeine and alcohol intake. Reduce your caffeine so you don't get withdrawal symptoms during the diet, such as headaches and grumpiness. During the programme, the only caffeine you will drink is white/ green tea. Three cups of white/green tea are equivalent to 1 cup of coffee or 2 cups of tea. If you regularly drink more than this quantity of tea and coffee, try and gradually cut down to one or two cups a day. You may also want to give white/green tea a try before you start the programme so you know what to expect.

The diet is alcohol free for three reasons: alcoholic drinks contain empty calories that we don't need; when we drink will-power tends to go out of the window so we eat more and finally, we sleep less well when we've been drinking. If you sleep less then you are more tired the next day, and a common side-effect of tiredness is to comfort eat. By cutting back on alcohol in the days leading up to the diet we are improving our sleep patterns and getting ourselves feeling good and ready to diet.

If you are doing the Lose a Stone in January programme as an accompaniment to Dry January (Dry January is total abstinence from alcohol for a month) then you should find they fit together perfectly. The "Lose a Stone" programme is designed to start on 4th January and last for 28 days, finishing on the 31st. If we work on the assumption that your last drink is on New Year's Eve (possibly into the very early hours of 1st January - I won't judge you if you don't judge me) then you've got 3 days to recover from New Year before the diet starts in earnest. If you've drunk enough over the Christmas period you won't miss it during the first half of January at all. And once you're passed half-way then the challenge is on and you won't want to let yourself down.

A few days before you start you need to think about what recipes you are going to cook in the first phase and purchase the necessary ingredients. You can then start preparing some of the meals in advance so you are ready to go.

A typical day

Start the day with a simple glass of water. Before you do anything else, pour yourself a nice cold glass of water (medium-sized is fine) and drink it before you think of tea, food or anything else. Why? Because you will always be dehydrated after sleep and any early morning hunger could be just a lack of water. It will help balance your body and will start to wake up your system more effectively than a cup of coffee or tea.

Next on the list is a cup of green or white tea. I know some of you will find this hard. For years and years I have always had a 'normal' cup of tea with milk to start the day and it is a bit of a shift. But, it's only for a month, it gets easier every day and, if you have prepared your body by reducing your tea and coffee intake in the week leading up to the diet, then you won't feel any caffeine withdrawal, just a light refreshing buzz from the small (but significant) amount of caffeine in the green tea.

Next...wait. Try to have your breakfast at least an hour after waking, but not more than 2½ hours. So if you get up at 7am, you should have breakfast between 8am and 9.30am. This is the optimum time because if you eat it too early, you won't have fully woken up and will not be properly hungry. You are in danger of getting hungrier earlier too. Likewise, if you have breakfast too long after getting up you will be famished and the breakfast won't fill you up, leaving you with possible cravings and the tendency to overeat later.

After your breakfast you should find that you are nicely full until lunchtime. But if you do feel yourself weakening, top up your white/green tea levels and that should give you a boost.

Lunch is often a relatively light meal, so make the most of it and savour the warmth and flavours. Make sure you drink a glass or two of water as well and finish off with a cup of white or green tea.

Dinner should be eaten relatively early, aim to eat between 5.30pm and 7.30pm as this is when your body needs it the most. Again, if possible, savour this meal. Take your time to prepare and serve it – don't just wolf it down. If you have other people's food to prepare as well, then I suggest making theirs first and eating yours in relative peace afterwards.

Finally, we reach the evening which, in truth, is the part of the day I struggle with the most. You've eaten all your food for the day, and the evening is distinctly lacking in excitement. It's often not a case of real hunger – more like boredom and habit. Many of us reach for whatever treats we can find in the evening and this is one of the most common causes of slow but steady weight-gain. The most important thing we can do is break this habit during the 28 days of the plan. It will get us a long way towards achieving our weight-loss goal and enable us to maintain the weight-loss when the programme is over.

Tips for evenings

- Be strict with yourself and remind yourself what it is all for.
- Distraction, distraction, distraction.
Keep away from the kitchen and wherever you hide

your treats. Watch TV, read a book, go to bed early.

- Stay active. Go for a walk & get some fresh air.

Keeping yourself hydrated

You need to say 'No' to diet drinks or anything with artificial sweeteners. We are trying to stick to real foods without chemical enhancement so rule these out for now.

Water and more water

I know it's boring but water is refreshing and good for you.

Sparkling water with ice and lemon

Make a glass of water so much more of an event by serving chilled sparkling mineral water over ice and lemon. This also works with still mineral water and even tap water.

Fresh lime soda

This is another way to jazz up a simple glass of water naturally. Place several ice cubes in a long tall glass. Halve a fresh lime and cut off one generous slice. Squeeze the rest of the lime juice into the glass. Add your choice of still or sparkling water and top with the slice of lime. This is extremely refreshing and virtually sugar-free so knock yourself out!

Fruit teas and more

Apart from the white/green tea that I am encouraging you to drink during the day, you may find a fruit tea, or a chamomile, peppermint or similar is just the ticket when you want something un-caffeinated and warming.

There are so many to choose from these days so stick to your favourite if you have one or try a selection if you're new to them.

A note about calorie counting

In previous books and on my blog www.52recipes.co.uk I have always included a calorie breakdown by portion for every recipe I create. The demand for the calorie information is so high that if I decide to leave out the calories for a new recipe I'll always get a request for the calorie count very soon. It's easy for me to count the calories in a recipe (after 5 calorie counted recipe books, I am like a walking calorie calculator!) so my desire to leave out the calorie information in this book is for very carefully thought out reasons. It is not without trepidation that I launch a book without calorie counts but it is with determination.

I have come to understand that counting calories is often counter-productive and leads us to make less healthy choices in the search for the lowest calorie count. Here are the simple facts - a calorie from fat is processed and used completely differently in the body from a calorie from carbohydrate. So why do we class them as the same? We all know that a fat contains more calories by weight than protein and that protein contains more calories by weight than carbohydrate. And what's the obvious result when we restrict our calories? We restrict our fat intake and increase our intake of empty carbs - often in the form of low fat 'health' foods containing lots of additives.

I know that for many people the need to count calories is an intrinsic part of any diet or weight-loss programme, so I'm not going to ask you to throw all of your trackers and calorie counters out of the window for good. All I'm asking is that you follow this programme for just 28 days - without counting calories - and see where it takes you.

The Ten Diet Steps

Every diet must have its rules and this one has ten guidelines to keep you on the straight and narrow.

1 **Drink green or white tea everyday**

   Try to drink at least 2 cups a day. Experiment with brands and flavours in the week before the diet as that will help you adjust.

2 **Don't drink alcohol**

   For the month of the diet you should cut out alcohol in your diet. Why? Think how even one small glass of wine might affect you. Firstly, is one glass ever enough? You relax and enjoy and suddenly your glass is empty. The temptation for a top-up is almost unavoidable. Secondly, any alcoholic drink will lower your resistance to extra foods and snacking. Be strict with yourself and don't allow a drop to pass your lips for the month long plan. If you break once, you'll feel like you've let yourself down and honestly, you'll end up giving up and breaking the alcohol ban and other weight-loss steps too. Consider it a challenge and reward yourself at the end - remember it's just a month. You can do this!

3 **Less red meat**

   Red meat is higher in saturated fat than chicken or fish. What's more the type of saturated fat found in red meat, especially processed red meat, has been proven to cause added stress to the body. Saturated fat found in dairy is better for you.

4   Fresh real ingredients

This weight-loss programme encourages healthy patterns that will help you keep the weight off with healthy 'real' recipes. Processed food is digested quicker and can leave you prone to unnecessary hunger.

5   No bread, pasta or other wheat based foods

Calories from bread and pasta are empty calories. They don't fill you up and you are soon hungry again. They are digested quicker than other carbohydrates and are more easily converted to fat cells. What's more, in many people, wheat can lead to bloating and digestive problems. Cut them out for the 28 days of the programme and see if you notice the difference.

6   Low sugar

Sugar or sweetened foods are harder to resist than others. You are naturally drawn to sweeter foods. But if you cut back to very little sugar then your sweet cravings will be reduced. After eating sugar, you might notice a sugar-high: a surge of energy as the sugar is turned into energy. But a high is always followed by a low. Within 2 hours of eating sugar, your body will be calling out for more food and more sugar. Break this cycle and you'll lose weight much quicker.

7   Cut caffeine

Coffee and tea are great. I love my morning cuppa – it's the best drink of the day. But our dependence on these drinks gets in the way of our diet goals. So for the month of the diet, the only caffeine should come in the form of green or white tea. If you're a caffeine addict you might suffer from a few withdrawals symptoms such as headaches and grumpiness. It is much easier to follow the programme if you cut down coffee and tea in the week before the diet.

8   Get enough sleep

Diet and weight-loss programmes are too often focussed on what you eat and how you exercise. The importance of a good night's sleep is frequently over-looked. When you don't get enough sleep levels of the hormone leptin drop, which increases appetite. The surge in appetite makes the wrong foods more appealing and easily derails your weight-loss effort. Not everyone needs a full 8 hours a night, but we could all do with getting to bed a little earlier. Think about when you normally go to bed and set yourself a goal of 15 minutes earlier. Separate yourself from your phone or devices at least an hour before bed. And consider a relaxing bath or snuggling up with a good book before bed.

9   Eat more citrus

Citrus fruits, particularly grapefruit, can help stimulate fat burning hormones. Half a grapefruit as part of your breakfast (not during your protein phases) can help lower insulin, a fat storage hormone, and that can assist your weight-loss. However, if you are on certain medicines, you should not have grapefruit so check the label or ask your doctor. If in doubt, swap the grapefruit for an orange. Never be tempted to swap the real thing for a juice, even if freshly squeezed, the sugar in the juice is always too high.

Another citrus-y treat is to squeeze half a lime or lemon into a glass of icy cold water - either still or sparkling - to make a refreshing change to plain water.

10 Get a daily dose of probiotics

Although a full understanding of how our gut bacteria is decades away, the importance of our gut health cannot be underestimated. As well as many other health benefits a good balance of gut bacteria seems to influence our ability to digest foods properly and therefore our overall food consumption. It doesn't need to be hard, a daily portion of natural live yogurt (not low fat) is all you need.

If you're not a fan of dairy, then a probiotic supplement is the answer. Look for supplements in a tablet or powder form and avoid the probiotic drinks as these have additives and sugar added. Remember with probiotics its very hard to see a definite change but know that they're secretly helping you. They normally take at least 3 weeks to see any effect so if you have any digestive issues see if they have improved over the course of the programme.

LIFESTYLE CHOICES

You now have all the diet and nutritional needs taken care of, so it's important to understand how other factors affect your body's fat burning abilities.

Your hormones are strongly affected by environmental factors such as sleep, caffeine, alcohol, hydration and stress. If you don't consider these factors then you will not be getting the most from your diet and exercise programme. Although you may not appreciate it yet, your choices regarding these factors are just as important as your decisions about food and exercise.

If you've wondered why you haven't made real progress even when eating super healthily and exercising well, then you must look at the choices you make in these areas and make adjustments. It's not rocket science and if you want sustained weight-loss as well as a healthier outlook on life then you've got to start here.

Sleep

A good night's sleep improves your mood, burns fat and slows the ageing process. When you consider that, is it really important to stay up late watching rubbish telly? Or is it just a habit that has become the norm? If you consider yourself to be a night-owl then a good proportion of this is down to your own training and reinforcement of bad habits. Reset them slowly, 10-15 minutes at a time and you'll get there.

Eight full hours of sleep is what you need to aim for, any less than this and you will be more tempted by snacks, especially sweet treats, the next day. Also in the later hours of the night, you'll start burning fat. If you only sleep for 6-7 hours you may not reach this zone and you'll still be burning last night's dinner!

So here are my 'sleep training' tips to get quality sleep. You'll be amazed by the effect on your mood and your weight.

1 **Start preparing for bed by 10pm at the latest**

   That means: TV off, devices away, bright lights turned off or dimmed.

2 **Relax**

   10-20 minutes of your bedtime routine should be dedicated to some 'you time'. You could read a book, listen to the radio, put on your favourite music, have a bath etc. The most important thing is to remove yourself from bright screens, get warm and cosy and turn off your brain. I love to read but also really like listening to drama or comedy through my DAB radio or the BBC radio app. The number of times I have drifted off to sleep listening to BBC Radio 4 extra is ridiculous!

Are our phones turning us into sleepless zombies?

This is what I used to do every night: 1. Go to plug my phone in. 2. Because my phone is in my hand, I'll just go and check facebook, my email, messages one more time. 3. Something totally unimportant catches my eye and I'll read it for 10 minutes. 4. I'll put my phone down without plugging it in. 5. Repeat from step 1!

If you think this is something that happens to you, you are not alone. Many of us are addicted to our little entertainment devices. And this is having an extremely negative effect on our sleep patterns.

So here's what you need to do: set a no phone time - 9pm, 9.30pm, definitely no later than 10pm. After this time DO NOT CHECK YOUR PHONE. Plug it in, forget about it. Don't go looking for those notifications that someone has liked your post (I do this all the time!), it can wait until the morning. My phone goes into 'night mode' where the screen changes from blue light to yellow light at 9.30pm. At that point, I know it's time to put it away. I allow myself one last check (but no dawdling) and then plug it in. If I go and check it after this I know I'm being very naughty so it helps to dissuade me.

3   Don't eat for at least 2 hours before bedtime

Let's be even more clear about this. Do not let any food pass your lips after 8pm. This is important for 2 reasons. Firstly, the late evening is when we tend to feel tempted. It's all too easy to grab a little something for a treat. And it's always sweet and bad for us. Whether it's chocolate, cake or biscuits, or body says it wants comfort and we are at our weakest in the evenings. It's not a hunger thing. You've eaten a good filling dinner, maybe even allowed yourself a little something sweet afterwards but your hand strays towards your secret stash of bad food before your brain realises what you are doing.

Best way to avoid it - remove it from the house. It's a rare night when you'll make the effort to go out to the nearest convenience store to buy yourself a treat. If you can't remove it from the house - most likely reason, kids or other family members require treats - then do what I do and make them store it in their bedrooms. We went to Cadbury World last week and came home with mountains of chocolate. I told the children that if they left it where I could find it then I WOULD eat it. They all squirrelled it away. Make sure they know that they're not allowed to eat it without your permission though!

4   **A herbal drink**

If you've got a hot herbal drink that you like, then warm and relax yourself with your favourite. Chamomile is good for sleep, but peppermint, roobios or any fruity non-caffeinated drink is lovely and relaxing. About 9pm is probably the time you want to settle down with a cup of your favourite.

Finally, a quick word for those of you who look at this and laugh 'well for X or Y reason, 8 hours sleep is never gonna happen' Maybe you've got babies, poorly children or have health problems that stop you getting a full night's sleep. For you a short nap in the afternoon will help enormously. Taking a 30 minute power nap or a longer 2 hours snooze will allow you to reset your hormone levels and control hunger and cravings. Naps don't make up for a good night's sleep but they are the next best thing.

Stress

Life is stressful. Everyone is different but we all have some stress in our lives. What if we could turn down our stress and eliminate some or all of it from our lives? Yes that's right we'd be healthier and leaner too. Ever gone to bed worrying about a problem that seems insurmountable but by morning, it seems tiny and not worth the bother? It's called making a mountain out of a molehill and we do it all the time. There is stress we can control and stress we can't and it all takes it's toll on our bodies.

We already have the tools to reduce our stress levels. But it is being aware of when we are over-stressed and making it our priority to deal with it when it starts to affect our mood or our sleep. Got too much work on and find yourself working late into the night. Stop. Give yourself a time limit and absolutely stop then. You will work faster and better the next day if you cut it out and get a good sleep. Worrying about your children, a friend or an argument. If there's nothing else you can do about it today, then make sure you switch it off along with your phone. Concentrate on something else - like a book or TV and allow yourself to relax. When you think about it in the morning it won't seem as bad and you may even have come up with the perfect solution while you slept.

SUGGESTED MEAL PLANS

Meal Plan: Detox and De-stress

The Detox and De-stress phase is for Days 1-4 of the course.

This is a suggested meal plan for those four days. Use the meal planner as a guide and an inspiration for this phase. Then take a look at the Recipe and Tips & Cheats chapters for Detox and De-stress and adapt the planner to make the perfect tailored menu for you. Don't forget that there are also recipes in other phases of the plan that are also suitable for Detox & De-stress. These will be clearly labelled and give you even more options.

Suggested Meal Plan: Detox and De-stress

	Day 1	Day 2	Day 3	Day 4
	Easy Microwave Porridge (page 68)	Chia Choc Granola with natural yogurt (page 67)	Easy Microwave Porridge (page 68)	Chia Choc Granola with natural yogurt (page 67)
	Chicken and Root Vegetable Broth (page 71)	Chicken and Root Vegetable Broth (page 71)	Vegetable Chilli (page 73)	Vegetable Chilli (page 73)
	Baked Salmon Salad (page 83)	Salad Nicoise (page 81)	Salad Nicoise (page 81)	Chicken Poached in White Wine (page 87)

Your Meal Plan: Detox and De-stress

	Day 1	Day 2	Day 3	Day 4

Meal Plan: Protein & Healthy Fats

There are three Proteins & Healthy Fats phases in the 28 day programme, each lasting 4 days. Protein & Healthy Fats Phases are Phase 2 (Days 5-8), Phase 4 (Days 13-16) and Phase 6 (Days 21-24).

This is a suggested meal plan for the Proteins & Healthy Fats phase. Use the meal planner as a guide and an inspiration for this phase. Then take a look at the Recipe and Tips & Cheats chapters for Protein & Healthy Fats and adapt the planner to make the perfect tailored menu for you. Don't forget that there are also recipes in other phases of the plan that are also suitable for Proteins & Healthy Fats. These will be clearly labelled and give you even more options.

If the meal plan works well for you in the first Proteins & Healthy Fats phase, then feel free to keep it for the later stages of the programme. Alternatively, you can keep your favourites and swap in some other recipes to replace the ones you weren't quite so keen on. Or go for a totally new mix...

Suggested Meal Plan: Proteins & Healthy Fats

	Day 1	Day 2	Day 3	Day 4
	Vanilla Quark with Berries (page 97)	Banana Pancakes (page 95)	Spanish Vegetable Tortilla (page 98)	Spanish Vegetable Tortilla (page 98)
	Feta Salad with Olives and Soft-boiled egg (page 101)	Herby Chicken Lunchbox (page 104)	Chorizo and Bean Stew (page 112)	Brie and Grape Lunchbox (page 103)
	Chinese-style Chicken with Pak Choi (page 117)	Fresh Saag Paneer (page 123)	Garlic Butter Chicken (page 127)	Garlic Butter Chicken (page 127)

Your Meal Plan: Proteins & Healthy Fats

	Day 1	Day 2	Day 3	Day 4

Meal Plan: Better Carbs

There are two Better Carbs phases in the 28 day programme, each lasting 4 days. Better Carbs Phases are Phase 3 (Days 9-12) and Phase 5 (Days 17-20).

This is a suggested meal plan for the Better Carbs phase. Use the meal planner as a guide and an inspiration for this phase. Then take a look at the Recipe and Tips & Cheats chapters for Better Carbs and adapt the planner to make the perfect tailored menu for you. Don't forget that there are also recipes in other phases of the plan that are also suitable for Better Carbs. These will be clearly labelled and give you even more options.

If the meal plan works well for you in the first Better Carbs phase, then feel free to keep it for the second stage of the programme. Alternatively, you can keep your favourites and swap in some other recipes to replace the ones you weren't quite so keen on. Or go for a totally new mix...

Suggested Meal Plan: Better Carbs

	Day 1	Day 2	Day 3	Day 4
	Everyday Oats (page 137)	Bircher Muesli (page 138)	Bircher Muesli (page 138)	Chia Choc Granola with natural yogurt (page 67)
	Mexican Chicken Soup (page 143)	Mexican Chicken Soup (page 143)	Spicy Sweet Potato Soup (page 151)	Spicy Sweet Potato Soup (page 151)
	Lightly Spiced Prawns with Vegetable Rice (page 159)	Peanut Butter and Lime Prawns (page 161)	Mediterranean Lamb Hotpot (page 169)	Mediterranean Lamb Hotpot (page 169)

Your Meal Plan: Better Carbs

	Day 1	Day 2	Day 3	Day 4

Balanced Eating

Balanced Eating is the final stage of the weight-loss programme - Days 25-28.

The Balanced Eating phase is a little different from the other stages of the diet, in that the goal is to round off your diet with some of your favourite recipes from the preceding phases and also prepare you for healthy eating and good habits into the future.

There is no meal plan or specific recipes for the Balanced Eating phase of the plan, instead all the recipes from ALL the previous phases of the programme (that's Detox and De-stress, Proteins and Healthy Fats and Better Carbs) are available to you. Ideally you should choose a mix with a few recipes from each phase but the choice is yours. Pick your favourites or try something new - every single recipe in this programme is healthy, balanced and good for you!

EXERCISE

We don't want to forget about exercise during this month. But also it is not our top priority. 80% of weight-loss comes from diet alone and actually stressing our bodies too much with intense exercise will leave us hungry and more likely to binge eat. This weight-loss plan works so well because we are decreasing the stress on our bodies and waking up our metabolism. But I'm not suggesting even for a moment that we give up on existing exercise routines or ignore exercise during the month.

Exercise when done right and in moderation helps us to build muscle and burn fat. Have a look at the three options and choose which best suits you at the present time. This means looking at yourself honestly and if you'd like to be a regular exerciser but are actually a sporadic or occasional exerciser then look at the occasional exercise routine. Maybe next time you check you'll be a regular exerciser.

Type of exercise, length of training and frequency of exercise are all key to a good balance. In a typical week you should look to only do 'sweaty' exercise a maximum of 3 times. The best kind of exercise to do during these sessions is strength or body weight training and/or high intensity (HIT) training. Strength training should be no more than an hour in duration and high intensity exercise no more than 30 minutes. You should also consider mixing in some less strenuous and relaxing exercises. Examples of these are yoga, pilates, swimming or walking.

If you are a regular exerciser...

You should consider yourself a regular exerciser if you do a higher intensity (sweaty) exercise 3 or more times a week. If your preferred exercise is cardio eg running, cycling, spin classes etc, then consider swapping up to 2 of these for a more strength based training if you can. Strength based training builds muscles and carries on burning fat for up to 48 hours after exercise. Whereas cardio burns more calories while exercising (less overall) and leaves you feeling depleted, hungry and more likely to eat food that you shouldn't.

As well as strength or HIT exercises - which you should aim to do every 2 days - you can intersperse these routines with more relaxing exercises. A gentle swim or walk can do wonders for your relaxation and well-being. Yoga and pilates are also fantastic for relaxation and toning your core.

If you are an occasional exerciser

You should consider yourself an occasional exerciser if on average you do some proper exercise about once a week. If that exercise is cardio, for example going for a run or an aerobics class, then please consider changing to something that is more strength based for this month only. If you want to continue with your class then perhaps you can add in something more strength based as well? Don't worry if you can't find something suitable, just be aware that although your exercise will improve your well-being it will also leave you hungry. So you will need to be careful that day. Most importantly of all you should add some non-strenuous exercise into your weekly routine. Gently exercise is relaxing and makes you feel great while still burning calories. The simplest of all is a half an hour walk. But a gentle swim or a yoga class would be perfect too. Ideally you should try to do non-strenuous exercise 3 times a week. If you don't believe this is helping you at all, rate your mood at 4pm on a day when you exercise and a day when you don't and I bet you'll see an improvement on an exercise day.

If you do not exercise

Never fear, I am not going to ask you to force you into lots of exercise with which you are uncomfortable. As I said before 80% of weight-loss is down to diet so changing your routine for this plan is not necessary. What I would suggest is that you do 30 minutes of walking at least 3 times a week. It would be even better if you tried to do this every day. Think about how or where you could do this. Is it getting off the bus at an earlier stop? A walk round the town at lunchtime? A stroll with the dog (or someone else's) at the end of the day? However you do it, the walk should be no less than 30 minutes long and at a brisk pace. In simple terms this means that you are exerting yourself but you can still carry on a conversation.

Why is simple walking so beneficial?

Walking is a fantastic exercise for many reasons. Perhaps the most important is that it lowers your stress hormones. This not only makes you feel better but also encourages your body to burn fat not sugar.

Your metabolic response to walking means that each time you walk (or swim or do yoga) you are reducing your insulin resistance by a tiny bit and enhancing your ability to burn fat. So never dismiss walking as 'not proper exercise', embrace and enjoy it.

RECIPES: DETOX AND DE-STRESS

Breakfast

Chia Choc Granola

Easy Microwave Porridge

Fruity Bran Loaf

Fruit Salad

Lunch

Chicken and Root Vegetable Broth

Vegetable Chilli (V)

French Country Salad (V)

Smoked Fish Chowder

Toasted Cumin Halloumi with Butternut Squash (V)

Mexican Beans and Cheese (V)

Dinner

Salad Niçoise

Baked Salmon Salad with Creamy Mint Dressing

Superfood Salad

Chicken Poached in White Wine

Breakfast

CHIA CHOC GRANOLA

This amazing recipe is an absolute diet staple. Clever use of ingredients mean that this recipe is more protein and fibre-rich than other cereals. And it contains only complex carbs and sugars. As a result, when combined with 100ml semi-skimmed milk or 100g natural yogurt this makes a really tasty and satisfying breakfast. Energy is released slowly and it is guaranteed to keep you full and curb hunger pangs for at least 4 hours. One batch makes seven 45g portions.

Suitable for: Detox and De-stress, Better Carbs

Serves 7 • Ready in 40 minutes

200g jumbo oats
20g flaked almonds
20g chia seeds
2 tbsp (30ml) mild olive oil
10g butter
1 heaped tbsp (40g) malt extract
40g dark chocolate chips

- Pre-heat the oven to 160C/140C fan. Line a large lipped baking tray with greaseproof paper or a silicone sheet.

- In a large mixing bowl, combine the oats, almonds and chia seeds.

- Place the olive oil, butter and malt extract in a small non-stick saucepan. Heat very gently, stirring until the butter has melted and the ingredients have combined. Do not allow to bubble or boil.

- Remove from the heat and pour into the oats. Mix together until all the oats have light coating of the sweet butter. When fully coated, tip out onto the prepared baking tray and distribute over the tray. Allow some gaps and a few clumps to form on the tray rather than an even spread. Bake in the pre-heated oven for 18-20 minutes.

- Remove from the oven and allow to cool completely on the tray. When cool, lightly break up larger pieces of granola. Sprinkle the chocolate chips over. Transfer to a lidded jar or air-tight container and store until needed.

EASY MICROWAVE PORRIDGE

This is my foolproof way of making great porridge.

Suitable for: Detox and De-stress, Better Carbs

SERVES 1 • Ready in 4 minutes

40g rolled oats
....
120ml semi-skimmed milk
....
100ml water
....

- Simply combine the oats, milk and water in a high-sided microwave-safe bowl or jug.

- Microwave on high power for 3 minutes. Stir thoroughly and add a little extra milk if necessary to gain the right consistency.

-

FRUITY BRAN LOAF

This fibre-rich loaf has no added sugar or sweetener. Lasts for about a week in an air-tight container. Serve with a generous spread of real butter or cream cheese.

Suitable for: Detox and De-stress

SERVES 8 • *Ready in 1 hr 30 mins (including soaking time)*

80g oat bran
100g sultanas
100g dried apricots, chopped
50g stoned dates, chopped
300ml milk (semi-skimmed or full-fat)
Butter for greasing
80g wholemeal flour
1 tsp baking powder
1 egg

- Place the oat bran and dried fruit in a bowl and pour over the milk. Stir and then leave to soak for at least 30 minutes.

- Preheat the oven to 180°C/160°C fan/350°F/gas mark 4. Grease a small loaf tin and line the base with baking parchment.

- In a large mixing bowl, combine the flour and baking powder.

- Whisk the egg into the milk and fruit mixture and then add this to the flour; stir well. You are looking for a gloopy dough so if the mixture feels too firm, add about 3 tablespoons of water. Scoop the mixture into the prepared loaf tin and bake for 40 minutes until golden brown on the top.

- Leave to cool completely before slicing. This loaf can be frozen as a whole or in individual slices.

FRUIT SALAD

This fruit salad makes a healthy light and flavoursome breakfast.

Suitable for: Detox and De-stress, Better Carbs

Serves 1 • Ready in 10 minutes

½ cup freshly made green tea
1 tsp honey
1 orange, halved
1 apple, cored and roughly chopped
10 red seedless grapes
10 blueberries

- Stir the honey into half a cup of green tea. When dissolved, add the juice of half the orange. Leave to cool.
- Chop the other half of the orange and place in a bowl together with the chopped apple, grapes and blueberries. Pour over the cooled tea and leave to steep for a few minutes before serving.

Lunch

CHICKEN AND ROOT VEGETABLE BROTH

This light and refreshing broth still provides a good source of protein in the chicken.

Suitable for: Detox and De-stress

Serves 2 • Ready in 2 hours

1 onion, peeled and roughly chopped
....
1 carrot, peeled and chopped
....
1 stick celery, trimmed and chopped
....
2 chicken drumsticks, skin on
....
1 litre water
....
8 whole peppercorns
....
1 tsp salt
....
1 bay leaf
....
1 small parsnip, peeled and finely chopped
....
1 small carrot, peeled and finely chopped
....
1 clove garlic, peeled and crushed
....
1 tbsp light soy sauce
....
2 tsp English mustard
....
2 spring onions, trimmed
and finely chopped
....
Pinch of freshly ground black pepper
....

- Take a large lidded pan and place the onion, carrot and celery inside. Add the peppercorns, salt and bay leaf.

- Pour in approximately 1 litre water and bring to a simmer. Place the lid on the pan and cook gently either on the hob or in a medium oven (170C fan) for 1½ hours. Add the chicken drumsticks for the last 30 minutes of cooking time.
- Strain the broth through a sieve. Discard the vegetables and place the chicken drumsticks on a plate. Leave to cool for 15 minutes or until the drumsticks can be handled comfortably.
- Return the broth to the pan. Add the parsnip, carrot and garlic to the broth and simmer for about 15 minutes until tender.
- Remove the skin from the drumsticks and pull the chicken off the bone. The chicken will just fall off the bone after its long cooking time. Discard the bones, skin and waste and separate the good chicken into 2 portions.
- Add the soy sauce, English mustard and spring onions to the broth and stir. Add the pepper and taste to check the seasoning. Divide the broth between 2 containers equally. Refrigerate the broth and the chicken separately until needed.
- When you are ready to eat the broth, reheat a portion until lightly bubbling. Then add the chicken and warm through.

VEGETABLE CHILLI (V)

This is a classic filling recipe that really sets you up for the whole day. The kidney beans add a little bit of protein and some good carbs so get stuck in and enjoy. This can be made in advance and chilled/frozen in individual portions so can be ready to eat in minutes.

Suitable for: Detox and De-stress, Better Carbs

Makes 3 portions • Ready in 45 minutes

300g chopped butternut squash (this is the cut weight and you can buy pre-prepared)
....
½ tsp ground cinnamon
....
2 tsp olive oil
....
1 red onion, peeled and chopped
....
1 green pepper, seeded and chopped
....
1 green chilli, seeded and sliced into rings
....
1 clove garlic, peeled and finely chopped
....
Zest and juice 1 lime
....
1 tsp mild chilli powder
....
1 tsp ground cumin
....
½ tsp paprika
....
½ tsp cocoa powder
....
1 tsp salt
....
1x 400g tin chopped tomatoes
....
1x400g tin kidney beans in water
....
Freshly ground pepper
....

• Preheat the oven to 220C/200C fan.

- Place the butternut squash on a baking tray, sprinkle over the cinnamon and season generously with salt and pepper. Drizzle over 1 tsp of olive oil and toss through with your hands. Bake in the oven for 15–20 minutes, until just tender.

- Meanwhile, heat the remaining teaspoon of olive oil in a large pan and add the onion, green pepper and chilli. Fry gently for 5 minutes. Add the garlic and lime zest and cook for a further minute or two. Add the chilli powder, cumin, paprika, cocoa powder and salt. Stir through before adding the chopped tomatoes and kidney beans (including the water).

- Bring up to a gentle simmer and cook, lid off, for about 30 minutes. Add the butternut squash and lime juice and stir through gently. Taste and add salt and pepper to taste. Cook for a further 5 minutes. Allow to cool completely (this allows the flavours to develop) before storing as three individual portions. Reheat on the hob or in the microwave before serving.

FRENCH COUNTRY SALAD (V)

The addition of the cannellini beans makes this a filling and hearty salad. The rest times are important to develop the best flavour of the salad.

Suitable for: Detox and De-stress, Better Carbs

Serves 2 • Ready in 15 minutes

1 sprig mint (5g), finely chopped
1 sprig basil (5g), finely chopped
1 tbsp extra virgin olive oil
Juice of 1 lemon
1 tsp Dijon mustard
Pinch of sugar
Salt and freshly ground black pepper
1 × 400g tin cannellini beans, rinsed and drained
1 red onion, chopped
1 large handful (20g) parsley, finely chopped
4 tomatoes, roughly chopped
½ cucumber, roughly cubed

- Place the chopped mint, basil, olive oil, lemon juice, mustard and sugar in a small bowl. Add a generous seasoning of salt and pepper. Leave to rest for 5 minutes.

- Place the cannellini beans, red onion, parsley, tomatoes and cucumber in a larger bowl. Pour over the dressing and stir to incorporate. Leave to rest for 5 minutes before serving.

SMOKED FISH CHOWDER

This is easy healthy comfort food and is perfect for warming you up.

Suitable for: Detox and De-stress, Better Carbs

Serves 4 • Ready in 40 minutes

10 black peppercorns
1 bay leaf
400g skinless smoked haddock or cod
500ml semi-skimmed milk
500ml fish or vegetable stock (fresh or made with 1 cube)
1 tsp olive oil
4 leeks, trimmed and cut into thin rings
½ tsp cumin seeds
500g new potatoes, skin on, quartered

- Place the peppercorns, bay leaf and fish in a saucepan. Pour in the milk and stock and bring to a gentle simmer. Continue to simmer gently until just cooked through, about 6–8 minutes. Remove the fish from the pan and set aside, reserving the cooking liquid.

- Meanwhile in a wide lidded frying pan (skillet), heat the oil over a low heat and stir in the leeks. Put the lid on and soften the leeks for 10 minutes.

- Remove the lid from the leeks and turn up the heat. Add the cumin seeds and fry until they start to sizzle and pop, then stir in the potatoes. Pour in the poaching liquid from the fish and bring to the boil. Reduce the heat and simmer for 15–20 minutes until the potatoes are tender.

- Turn off the heat. Break the fish apart gently with your fingers and add to the soup. Heat gently for 1–2 minutes before serving.

TOASTED CUMIN HALLOUMI WITH BUTTERNUT SQUASH (V)

This unusual dish has a North African feel to it, with the touch of heat tempered by the sweetness of the butternut squash and the saltiness of the halloumi.

Suitable for: Detox and De-stress, Better Carbs

SERVES 2 • *Ready in 15 minutes*

300g (½ small) butternut squash, peeled and cut into large chunks
1 tsp cumin seeds
1 tsp chilli flakes
1 tbsp rapeseed oil
2 tsp tomato purée
1 tsp garlic purée (or 1 clove, crushed)
120g halloumi, cut into chunks
1 spring onion, trimmed and chopped
50g piquante peppers from a jar, drained and chopped
Juice of 1 lime
Freshly ground black pepper
Handful of fresh coriander, chopped (optional)

- Place the cubed butternut squash into a microwaveable dish, cover and microwave for 5 minutes on high. Place a frying pan over a medium/high heat and toss in the cumin seeds and chilli flakes. Dry fry for one minute, then reduce the heat to medium and add the oil, tomato purée and garlic. Stir for a few seconds before adding the halloumi and spring onions. Stir-fry for 3 minutes.

- Add the peppers and butternut squash and continue to cook, stirring regularly, until browned on all sides. Remove from the heat and stir in the lime juice, black pepper and coriander. Serve immediately.

MEXICAN BEANS AND CHEESE (V)

These beans add a bit of pizzazz to lunchtime. As the flavour improves with time, you can leave some spare for another day; it will keeps well in the fridge for 2–3 days.

Suitable for: Detox and De-stress, Better Carbs

SERVES 2 • Ready in 5 mins

1 x 400g tin kidney beans,
rinsed and drained
....
1 tsp mild chilli powder
....
½ tsp ground cumin
....
1 tsp dried oregano
....
2 handfuls of crisp lettuce, such
as iceberg or little gem
....
2 medium tomatoes, roughly chopped
....
40g Cheddar cheese, grated
....
Salt and freshly ground black pepper
....

- Tip the drained beans into a shallow bowl and roughly mash with the back of a fork. Sprinkle over the chilli powder, cumin, oregano and a generous sprinkling of salt and pepper. Mix together until thoroughly combined.
- Arrange the lettuce leaves on a plate and top with a generous serving of the beans. Add the tomatoes and finally the grated cheese.

Dinner

SALAD NIÇOISE

You can't beat a traditional ... ish Salad Niçoise.

Suitable for: Detox and De-stress, Better Carbs

Serves 2 • Ready in 40 minutes

200g new potatoes, quartered
50g fresh or frozen soya/edamame beans
2 large eggs
4 large tomatoes, roughly chopped
10cm piece (150g) cucumber, halved lengthways and sliced
½ red pepper, thinly sliced
50g good-quality black olives, pitted
1 tbsp capers, rinsed and drained
4 anchovy fillets, cut into thin slices
Large handful (20g) parsley, roughly chopped
For the dressing:
1 clove garlic, peeled
2 anchovies, roughly chopped
3–4 basil leaves
Salt and freshly ground black pepper
2 tbsp extra virgin olive oil
1 tsp red wine vinegar

- Steam the new potatoes for 15–20 minutes until just tender. Adding the soya beans for the last 4 minutes if frozen, or the last minute if fresh. Leave to cool.

- Prick the eggs and lower into a pan of boiling water. Boil for 9 minutes. Remove and place in a pan of cold water for a few minutes before peeling and quartering.

- To make the dressing, use a food processor, coffee grinder or pestle and mortar to grind together the garlic, anchovies, basil leaves and salt and pepper. Stir in the olive oil and vinegar.

- Put the tomato, cucumber, red pepper, olives, capers, anchovies and parsley in a large bowl with the potatoes and soya beans. Mix lightly to combine, add the dressing then mix again. Arrange the quartered eggs over the top just before serving.

BAKED SALMON SALAD WITH CREAMY MINT DRESSING

Baking the salmon in the oven makes this salad so simple.

Suitable for: Detox and De-stress, Proteins and Healthy Fats

Serves 1 • Ready in 20 minutes

1 salmon fillet (130g)

40g mixed salad leaves

40g young spinach leaves

2 radishes, trimmed and thinly sliced

5cm piece (50g) cucumber, cut into chunks

2 spring onions, trimmed and sliced

1 small handful (10g) parsley,
roughly chopped

For the dressing:

1 tsp low-fat mayonnaise

1 tbsp natural yogurt

1 tbsp rice vinegar

2 leaves mint, finely chopped

Salt and freshly ground black pepper

- Preheat the oven to 200°C (180°C fan/Gas 6).
- Place the salmon fillet on a baking tray and bake for 16–18 minutes until just cooked through. Remove from the oven and set aside. The salmon is equally nice hot or cold in the salad. If your salmon has skin, simply cook skin side down and remove the salmon from the skin using a fish slice after cooking. It should slide off easily when cooked.

- In a small bowl, mix together the mayonnaise, yogurt, rice wine vinegar, mint leaves and salt and pepper together and leave to stand for at least 5 minutes to allow the flavours to develop.
- Arrange the salad leaves and spinach on a serving plate and top with the radishes, cucumber, spring onions and parsley. Flake the cooked salmon onto the salad and drizzle the dressing over.

SUPERFOOD SALAD

This delicious salad combines chicken with vegetables, nuts and seeds to get as much healthy goodness as you can in a bowl.

Suitable for: Detox and De-stress, Proteins and Healthy Fats

SERVES 1 • *Ready in 20 minutes*

10g whole almonds
10g cashews
10g sunflower seeds
10g pomegranate seeds
1 tsp olive oil
1 small chicken fillet (100g), skinless and boneless, cut into thin strips
2 tsp soy sauce
½ tsp honey
¼ tsp ground ginger
5 florets (40g) of broccoli
Handful (40g) of sugar snap peas
50g mixed salad leaves
1 fresh mint leaf, finely chopped (optional)
Small bunch (10g) of flat-leaf parsley, finely chopped (optional)
1 tomato, roughly chopped
1 spring onion, chopped

- Place a small dry frying pan over a medium heat until toasty hot. Toss in the almonds, cashews and seeds. Dry fry for a few minutes, stirring frequently, until they release their aromas and start to brown. Remove from the pan and set aside.

- Add the olive oil and chicken strips to the still hot pan. Fry the chicken for 8-10 minutes, until cooked through. Remove from the pan and set aside. Meanwhile, prepare the honey dressing for the chicken. In a shallow bowl, mix together the soy sauce, honey and ginger. Stir the chicken into the dressing. Leave to rest while you prepare the rest of the salad. Simmer the broccoli and sugar snap peas together for approximately 6 minutes until tender.

- Arrange the mixed leaves, herbs (if using), tomato and spring onions on a serving plate or bowl. Add the broccoli and sugar snaps. Arrange the chicken over the top and sprinkle on the nuts and seeds. Finally drizzle over any remaining dressing.

CHICKEN POACHED IN WHITE WINE

Serve with basmati rice and broccoli.

Suitable for: Detox and De-stress, Better Carbs

Serves 1 • Ready in 20 minutes

1 tsp olive oil
....
½ garlic clove, peeled and crushed
....
2 spring onions, trimmed and sliced
....
½ tsp dried mixed herbs
....
1 × 150g skinless chicken breast, halved
....
100ml dry white wine
....
1 tbsp soft cheese
....
small handful of fresh parsley, chopped
....

- Heat the oil, garlic, spring onions and dried mixed herbs in a small lidded frying pan or saucepan for 1–2 minutes until sizzling. Add the chicken and cook for about 4 minutes until the first side turns golden.

- Turn the chicken over and add the white wine. Put the lid on and turn the heat to low. Let the chicken continue to cook in the wine for a further 5 minutes. Check that the chicken is cooked through before removing from the pan and covering.

- Bring the remaining liquid in the pan back up to simmering and stir in the soft cheese. Bubble for 2–3 minutes until you get a pleasingly thick sauce. Stir in the parsley and pour over the chicken.

TIPS & TRICKS: DETOX AND DE-STRESS

We all know that sometimes there aren't enough hours in the day and sometimes cooking a healthy meal from scratch isn't an option. So here are some ideas for quick food to grab that is suitable for this stage of the plan. They're not meant for every meal of every day but if you get stuck you'll know what to grab.

Don't forget that during the Detox and De-stress phase you are allowed fruit. One portion with every meal is perfect. I wouldn't recommend banana (except as a main breakfast option) but berries, cherries, citrus fruits like orange or satsuma, apples, pears, kiwis are all good. It is much better to have fruit with or just after a meal rather than as a snack. BUT if you get desperate then one piece of fruit per day as a snack is acceptable.

Breakfast

- Banana
- Any oat-based cereal.

The less added sugar and extra ingredients the better. Also rolled oats are better than the smaller oat flakes. Granola and porridge are both fine. Try to avoid anything with low fat or fat free yogurt or milk.

- Natural yogurt sweetened with a smidge of jam. Again avoid low fat yogurts with any added ingredients.

Lunch

- A good quality soup

Obviously home-made is best but a fresh soup (ie not tinned) from a trusted brand is a good lunch choice for this phase. To make it more filling, you should choose one with lentils or beans. If you have a tomato soup or one thickened with potato then you are in danger of getting hungry late afternoon. Also check the ingredients list, a fresh soup shouldn't have any additives or ingredients you haven't heard of.

Dinner

If you cook nothing else for yourself, dinner is the one meal you should try and cook. A 'ready meal' of any variety just doesn't cut the mustard here. Your dinner should consist of quality protein (chicken or fish), good carbs (basmati rice, new potatoes in their skins) plus plenty of vegetables.

If you don't fancy any of the recipes, then grilled chicken or salmon fillet with new potatoes and broccoli would be an acceptable substitute. I promise that one of the detox and de-stress recipes would be more exciting though. If you don't fancy any of the recipes in this phase, remember that some of the dinner recipes from 'Better Carbs' are also acceptable.

RECIPES: PROTEINS AND HEALTHY FATS

Breakfast

Banana Pancakes

Smoked Salmon Rolls

Vanilla Quark with Berries

Spanish Vegetable Tortilla

Continental Plate

Home-made Beans

Lunch

Feta Salad with Olives and Soft-boiled Egg (V)

Brie and Grape Salad Lunchbox (V)

Herby Chicken Lunchbox

Feta Stuffed Red Peppers (V)

Egg Florentine (V)

LA Green Salad (V)

Sausages and Puy Lentils

Serrano Ham Salad

Chorizo and Bean Stew

Greek Salad Plate (V)

Dinner

Smoked Salmon & Soft-boiled Egg on Spinach and Cucumber Salad

Chinese-style Chicken with Pak Choi

Chicken Cassoulet

Moroccan Spiced Eggs (V)

Fresh Saag Paneer (V)

Creamy Baked Salmon with Mange Tout

Spanish Baked Prawns

Garlic Butter Chicken

Sesame Chicken Salad

Roast Chicken and Peanuts

Japanese Noodle Salad

Breakfast

BANANA PANCAKES

These are super simple pancakes with just two
ingredients - you guessed it bananas and egg. Really
tasty and easy to rustle up.

Suitable for: Proteins and Healthy Fats

Serves 1 • Ready in 10 minutes

1 banana
2 eggs
1 tsp mild olive oil

- Use the back of a fork to thoroughly mash the banana.

- In a separate bowl, whisk the eggs. Add the banana to the whisked eggs.

- Heat the oil in a medium frying pan until hot but not smoking. Pour in the pancake mix. Cook for 3-4 minutes, turning if you dare until just cooked but still a little wobbly.

SMOKED SALMON ROLLS

These parcels need a little preparation, but they can be made the night before and refrigerated.

Suitable for: Proteins and Healthy Fats

Serves 1 (makes 2 parcels) • Ready in 10 minutes

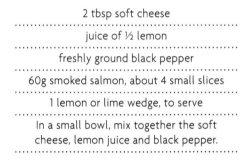

2 tbsp soft cheese

juice of ½ lemon

freshly ground black pepper

60g smoked salmon, about 4 small slices

1 lemon or lime wedge, to serve

In a small bowl, mix together the soft cheese, lemon juice and black pepper.

• Lay two pieces of salmon out in a cross shape, then place a large dollop of the cream cheese mixture in the middle of the cross. Bring up the sides of the salmon, twist slightly and stick a cocktail stick (toothpick) through the top. Make another parcel in the same way. Serve with a wedge of lemon or lime on the side.

VANILLA QUARK WITH BERRIES

A fresh and simple way to start the day. Quark is a great protein-rich alternative to yogurt.

Suitable for: Proteins and Healthy Fats

SERVES 1 • *Ready in 1 minute*

100g quark
1 tsp vanilla bean paste
1 tsp elderflower cordial
1 tbsp water
handful fresh or frozen berries

• Simply mix the ingredients together and serve.

SPANISH VEGETABLE TORTILLA

If you think eggs are worth a try for breakfast but don't want to be cooking and prepping first thing in the morning, a tortilla is a very good bet. The eggs are cooked slowly with vegetables and then left to cool before cutting into slices. Stick it in the fridge overnight and it will be ready and waiting for: a filling and perfectly balanced breakfast.

Suitable for: Proteins and Healthy Fats

Serves 2 • Ready in 30 minutes

1 tsp olive oil

1 small onion, roughly chopped

½ red pepper, roughly chopped

½ green pepper, roughly chopped

4 large eggs

4 cherry tomatoes, halved

Salt and freshly ground black pepper

- Heat the oil in a small, lidded frying pan over a medium/high heat. Toss in the onion and peppers and season generously with salt and pepper. Cook over a medium heat until sizzling and then stir, reduce the heat to low and place the lid (or a suitably sized plate) on top. Cook for a further 10 minutes until soft. Remove the vegetables from the pan and set aside.

- Whisk the eggs together in a bowl or jug and pour into the frying pan. After a couple of minutes, use a plastic spatula or fish slice to lift up the cooked edge of the eggs and allow the uncooked egg to run underneath. Continue to do this all round the pan.

Then return the cooked vegetables to the pan, add the tomatoes and put the lid on. Cook for around 10 minutes, or until the eggs in the centre are just firm.

- Flip the tortilla over on to a plate and leave to cool completely before cutting into quarters or wedges. The tortilla will keep for 48 hours in the fridge.

CONTINENTAL PLATE

Sometimes a good breakfast is all about presentation. This cold plate of meat and cheese is both filling and appetising. This is a great alternative to a greasy fry-up when you want to avoid carbs at breakfast.

Suitable for: Proteins and Healthy Fats

SERVES 1 • Ready in 10 mins

1 large egg

....

2 crisp lettuce leaves, such as little gem 1 tomato, quartered

....

1 chunky slice of good-quality ham, cut into 4 pieces

....

2 thick slices (30g) Gouda cheese

....

- First lightly boil your egg by placing it gently into a pan of simmering water. Cook for 7–9 minutes, depending on how you like it cooked. Remove from the pan with a slotted spoon and cool for a few minutes before peeling and cutting into quarters.
- Arrange the lettuce and tomatoes over one side of the plate, with the ham and cheese arranged on the other side. Finally place the quartered egg in the centre.

HOME-MADE BEANS

These have no added sugar or sweeteners and are really quick to make. I'm pretty sure you won't go back to shop-bought beans after trying these ones. Serve with a slice of grilled bacon and/or a scrambled egg.

Suitable for: Proteins and Healthy Fats, Better Carbs

SERVES 2 • Ready in 7 minutes

1 tsp olive oil

1 tbsp tomato purée

½ tsp Worcestershire sauce

250ml water

1 x 400g tin haricot beans, drained

2 tbsp red wine vinegar

1 tbsp maple syrup

1 tsp soy sauce

- Heat the oil in a pan over a low heat. Add the tomato purée and fry for a minute before adding the Worcestershire sauce, water and drained beans.

- Increase the heat and bring to a simmer before adding the red wine vinegar, maple syrup and tamari. Cook gently over a low heat for 5 minutes.

- Serve immediately or allow to cool and refrigerate (these beans only improve in flavour) for up to 2 days. Simply re-heat gently before serving.

Lunch

FETA SALAD WITH OLIVES AND SOFT-BOILED EGG (V)

A perfect egg with a slightly runny yolk makes you feel rather special...

Suitable for: Proteins and Healthy Fats

Serves 1 • Ready in 10 minutes

1 large egg
2 tsp extra virgin olive oil
½ tsp English mustard
pinch of sugar
1 tsp mayonnaise
juice of half lemon
salt and pepper
40g baby leaf spinach
5cm cucumber, halved lengthways and sliced
40g feta cheese, cut into small cubes or lightly crumbled
4 black olives, halved

- Heat a small pan of water to boiling. Using a slotted spoon, slowly lower the egg into the boiling water. Heat for 8-10 minutes depending on how well-cooked you like your egg. Remove from the water using the slotted spoon and cool in a bowl of cold water for a minute or two to stop the cooking process.

- Meanwhile, make the dressing by combining the olive

oil, mustard, sugar, mayonnaise, lemon juice and salt and pepper in a small bowl.

- Arrange the spinach and cucumber over a plate and pour over half the dressing. Add the feta and olives. Peel the just cooled egg and quarter. Arrange the egg pieces over the salad. Drizzle the rest of the dressing over. Serve immediately.

BRIE AND GRAPE SALAD LUNCHBOX (V)

This is a lunchbox salad as it can easily be prepared in the morning and transported in a container to your place of work. The salad and dressing can be made up separately and then combined at lunchtime. A small pot with a secure lid is perfect for the dressing - try re-using one from a store bought salad.

Suitable for: Proteins and Healthy Fats

Serves 1 • Ready in 5 minutes

50g baby kale

50g (5cm) cucumber, halved lengthways and sliced

Small handful (10g) flat-leaf parsley, leaves only

30g Brie, cut into chunks

About 10 red seedless grapes, halved

20g walnuts, halved

For the dressing:

1 tsp sesame oil

1 tsp extra virgin olive oil

Juice of 1/2 lime

1/2 tsp brown sugar

1/2 tsp salt

- Simply place the kale, cucumber and parsley on a serving plate or in a lunchbox. Arrange the Brie, grapes and walnuts over the top.

- Place all the dressing ingredients in a small dish (or lidded pot) and mix together. When you are ready to serve the salad, pour the dressing over.

HERBY CHICKEN LUNCHBOX

Make the dressing in a small lidded container and drizzle over the salad at lunchtime.

Suitable for: Proteins and Healthy Fats

Serves 1 • Ready in 5 minutes

50g fresh or frozen soya/edamame
beans 50g watercress leaves

....

Small handful (10g) flat-leaf
parsley, leaves only

....

1/4 red onion, cut into very thin slices

....

1 small roasted chicken breast
fillet (100g), sliced

....

For the dressing:

....

2 tsp extra virgin olive oil

....

Juice of 1/2 lemon

....

Pinch of sugar

....

2 leaves parsley, finely chopped

....

2 leaves basil, finely chopped

....

2 leaves mint, finely chopped

....

Salt and freshly ground black pepper

....

- If the soya beans are frozen or require cooking, cook as per the packet instructions and leave to cool.

- Arrange the watercress, edamame, parsley and red onion in a serving dish or lunchbox container. add the chicken.

- Mix together the olive oil, lemon juice, sugar, parsley, basil and mint in a small bowl or container. season generously with salt and pepper. Drizzle over the salad just before serving.

FETA STUFFED RED PEPPERS (V)

Suitable for: Proteins and Healthy Fats, Better Carbs

Serves 1 • Ready in 20 minutes

1 red pepper, top removed, halved and deseeded
1 tsp olive oil
½ x 400g can cannellini beans
½ clove garlic, crushed
Juice of half a lemon
Salt and pepper
1 spring onion, finely chopped
4 cherry tomatoes, roughly chopped
Small handful fresh parsley, stalks removed and finely chopped
40g feta cheese
4 black olives, sliced
40g baby spinach, stalks removed
5cm cucumber, halved and cut into semi-circles

- Preheat the oven to 240C/220C fan.
- Rub the red pepper halves all over with the olive oil. Place face down on a small baking tray and bake in the oven for 10 minutes.
- Meanwhile, place the cannellini bean, garlic and lemon juice in a small bowl. Mash the beans roughly with the back of a fork and stir until well-combined. Season with salt and pepper. Stir in the spring onion, cherry tomatoes and parsley.
- Remove the peppers from the oven and turn them

the right way up. Distribute the bean salad evenly between the two peppers. Crumble the feta over the top and add the olives. Return to the oven for a further 10 minutes.

- Serve the stuffed peppers straight from the oven on a bed of spinach leaves and cucumber.

EGG FLORENTINE (V)

A lovely quick meal for one.

Suitable for: Proteins and Healthy Fats

Serves 1 • Ready in 10 minutes

1 large egg
1 tbsp thick mayonnaise
¼ tsp Dijon mustard
Juice of ½ lemon
1 tsp extra virgin olive oil
Pinch of salt
¼ tsp ground turmeric
¼ tsp cayenne pepper
1 tsp capers
1 tsp (5g) butter
¼ tsp nutmeg
50g fresh spinach, stalks removed
Pinch of paprika

- Fill a shallow saucepan with 4–5cm water. Bring to a gentle simmer. Crack the egg on the side of the pan and lower slowly into the water. Simmer for exactly 1 minute. Turn off the heat and leave to cook in the slowly cooling water for a further 9 minutes. This should ensure a cooked egg with a runny middle.

- Next prepare the mock hollandaise. Mix the mayonnaise, mustard, lemon juice, olive oil, salt, turmeric and cayenne in a small bowl until smooth. Stir in the capers.

- In a small lidded pan, heat the butter and nutmeg

until the butter is just starting to sizzle. Add the spinach and stir through for 30 seconds. Then place the lid on the pan, turn off the heat and allow the spinach to wilt for 2 minutes.

• To serve, place the wilted spinach on a small plate, use a slotted spoon to remove the egg carefully from the water and place on top of the spinach. Pour over the hollandaise sauce and top with a pinch of paprika.

LA GREEN SALAD (V)

Suitable for: Proteins and Healthy Fats

Serves 2 • Ready in 15 minutes

100g small broccoli florets
100g asparagus, trimmed
50g watercress leaves
50g spinach leaves
200g ready-to-eat or cooked puy lentils
½ ripe avocado, stoned, peeled and cut into large chunks
20g pomegranate seeds
For the dressing:
2 tsp extra virgin olive oil
¼ tsp ground cumin
¼ tsp ground turmeric
Zest and juice of 1 lemon (washed in hot soapy water to remove wax first)
2 tbsp natural yogurt

- Steam the broccoli over a pan of boiling water for 5 minutes or until just tender. Add the asparagus for the last 2–4 minutes (2 minutes for 'al dente'). Leave to cool.

- Make the dressing by combining the olive oil, cumin, turmeric, lemon zest and juice with the natural yogurt in a small bowl.

- Toss together the watercress and spinach leaves with the broccoli, asparagus, lentils and avocado. Add the dressing and combine gently. Divide between two serving plates and serve with the pomegranate seeds sprinkled over.

SAUSAGES AND PUY LENTILS

This is a beautifully filling dish. The lentils have some carbohydrate but is such a good source of protein that this dish is included here. I use a pack of ready-to-eat puy lentils here to make the meal super easy to prepare. Make sure you use sausages that have already been cooked here.

Suitable for: Proteins and Healthy Fats

Serves 2 • Ready in 8 minutes

2 tsp olive oil
....
100g mushrooms, washed and sliced
....
2 spring onions, trimmed and chopped
....
2 good quality cooked
pork sausages, sliced
....
4 med tomatoes, roughly chopped
....
250g cooked puy lentils
....
Few drops worcestershire sauce
....

- Heat the oil on a high heat in a wide saucepan. Toss in the mushrooms and stir-fry until just cooked and tender. Add the spring onions and sausages and cook for a further 2-3 minutes until warmed. Still on a high heat, add the tomatoes and cook for 2 minutes.

- Finally add the puy lentils and worcestershire sauce and stir through until warmed. Season with a little salt and pepper and serve immediately.

SERRANO HAM SALAD

The sweetness of the blackcurrants beautifully offsets the saltiness of the ham and olives.

Suitable for: Proteins and Healthy Fats

Serves 1 • Ready in 5 minutes

40g baby kale

40g young spinach leaves

Small handful (10g) parsley, stalks discarded and roughly chopped

2 slices (30g) serrano ham, chopped

About 12 pitted Kalamata olives, halved

Handful (30g) blackcurrants, washed and stalks removed

For the dressing:

1 tsp capers, drained

1 tsp extra virgin olive oil

Juice of ½ lemon

Salt and freshly ground black pepper

- Combine the capers, olive oil, lemon juice and salt and pepper in a small bowl and set aside.
- Mix the kale, spinach and parsley lightly in a serving dish. Arrange the serrano ham, olives and blackcurrants over the top. Pour over the dressing and serve immediately.

CHORIZO AND BEAN STEW

This recipe takes less than ten minutes to cook and is wonderfully filling. For the mixed beans, I prefer to use kind that come vacuum-packed and ready to eat although tinned beans work just as well; just rinse and drain well before using.

Suitable for: Proteins and Healthy Fats

Serves 1 • Ready in 10 minutes

20g chorizo, finely chopped

150g ready-to-eat mixed beans (drained weight)

1 tbsp tomato purée

½ tsp chilli flakes

1 tsp red wine vinegar

Few drops Worcestershire sauce

50-75ml water

1 tbsp chopped fresh flat-leaf parsley, to garnish

- Place a small frying pan over a high heat until hot. Add the chopped chorizo and fry until turning brown on all sides, about 1–2 minutes.
- Reduce the heat to low and then add in the beans, tomato purée, chilli flakes, vinegar, Worcestershire sauce and water. Stir well to combine. Allow the stew to start bubbling gently and then cook for another 5 minutes, stirring occasionally. Serve immediately, garnished with chopped parsley.

GREEK SALAD PLATE (V)

When I want to feel a little bit special at lunchtime, I pull together some of my favourite ingredients to make this elegant yet quick dish.

Suitable for: Proteins and Healthy Fats

SERVES 1 • Ready in 5 mins

40g mixed salad leaves
....
1 tomato, roughly chopped
....
30g feta cheese, cut into generous cubes
....
8 large black olives
....
Generous dollop of houmous
....
Drizzle of extra-virgin olive oil
....
Drizzle of balsamic vinegar
....
Handful (20g) of pine nuts
....

- Take a large plate and arrange your salad leaves over one half. Arrange the tomato and feta over the leaves.

- Take two very small bowls or cups (try egg cups or espresso cups) and place your olives in one and your houmous in another and place on the plate. Drizzle the olive oil and balsamic vinegar over the salad and finally scatter over the pine nuts.

Dinner

SMOKED SALMON & SOFT-BOILED EGG ON SPINACH AND CUCUMBER SALAD

This dish is simple to throw together and is stack full or protein to fill you up. Smoked salmon gives it a luxurious feel.

Suitable for: Proteins and Healthy Fats

Serves 1 • Ready in 10 minutes

1 large egg
....
2 tsp extra virgin olive oil
....
½ tsp English mustard
....
pinch of sugar
....
1 tsp mayonnaise
....
juice of half lemon
....
salt and pepper
....
40g baby leaf spinach
....
5cm cucumber, halved
lengthways and sliced
....
60g smoked salmon, cut
into small thin slices
....

- Heat a small pan of water to boiling. Using a slotted spoon, slowly lower the egg into the boiling water. Heat for 8-10 minutes depending on how well-cooked you like your egg. Remove from the water using the slotted spoon and cool in a bowl of cold water for a minute or two to stop the cooking process.

- Meanwhile, make the dressing by combining the olive oil, mustard, sugar, mayonnaise, lemon juice and salt and pepper in a small bowl.
- Arrange the spinach and cucumber over a plate and pour over half the dressing. Add the salmon. Peel the just cooled egg and quarter. Arrange the egg pieces over the salmon. Drizzle the rest of the dressing over. Serve immediately.

CHINESE-STYLE CHICKEN WITH PAK CHOI

This delicious and filling stir-fry is perfect for the end of day two. You need a treat and this is perfect. It's really satisfying and will fill your kitchen with amazing smells.

Suitable for: Proteins and Healthy Fats

Serves 1 • Ready in 20 minutes

1 small skinless chicken breast (125g), cut into strips
....
1 tsp cornflour
....
1 tsp water
....
1 tsp rice wine
....
1 tsp tomato puree
....
½ tsp brown sugar
....
1 tbsp light soy sauce
....
½ clove garlic, peeled and grated
....
½ thumb (2cm) fresh ginger, peeled and grated
....
1 tsp olive oil
....
½ tsp walnut oil
....
50g shiitake mushrooms, sliced
....
2 spring onions, trimmed and shredded
....
100g pak choi, cut into thin slices
....
30g beansprouts
....

• Toss the chicken pieces in the cornflour until they are fully coated. Set aside. In a small bowl, stir together the water, rice wine, tomato puree, brown sugar and soy sauce. Add the garlic and ginger and stir together.

- In a wok or large frying pan, heat the olive and walnut oils together on a medium heat. Add the chicken and stir-fry for 4-5 minutes each side until cooked through. Remove the chicken from the pan with a slotted spoon and set aside.

- Turn the heat up to high, add the shiitake mushrooms to the pan and stir-fry for 2-3 minutes until cooked and glossy. Then add the spring onions, pak choi and beansprouts and stir-fry until the pak choi has wilted.

- Reduce the heat to low, then stir in the cooked chicken. Add the sauce and allow the sauce to bubble around the chicken for a minute. Remove from the heat and serve immediately.

CHICKEN CASSOULET

This is a great 'all-in-one' dish.

Suitable for: Proteins and Healthy Fats, Better Carbs

Serves 2 • Ready in 1 hour

1 tsp olive oil

2 shallots, peeled, halved and thinly sliced

1 small carrot, peeled and sliced

1 celery stick, trimmed and chopped

1 clove garlic, peeled and crushed

1 x 400g can chopped tomatoes

100ml red wine

300ml water

1 tsp dried thyme

2 tsp malt extract

½ tsp mild chilli powder

½ tsp smoked paprika

1 tsp salt

1 tsp walnut oil

1 bay leaf

1 x 400g can butterbeans in water

2 tsp (10g) butter

1 large or 2 small skinless chicken breasts
(approx. 200g total), cut into cubes

- Add the shallots, carrot and celery to the pan, stir, replace the lid and cook gently for 5-8 mins until soft. Add the garlic, chopped tomatoes, red wine, water, thyme, malt extract, chilli powder, smoked paprika, salt, walnut oil and bay leaf.

Bring to a simmer and cook with the lid ajar for about 30 minutes. Add the butterbeans and leave to cool if you don't want to eat immediately.

- When you are ready to serve the cassoulet: Warm through the cassoulet until just bubbling.
- Heat half the butter in a frying pan. When the butter has melted, add half the chicken and fry for approx. 2 mins each side until golden brown but not cooked through. Add the chicken to the cassoulet. Bring to simmering point again and cook for 8-10 minutes or until the chicken is just cooked and tender. Remove the bay leaf before serving.

MOROCCAN SPICED EGGS (V)

This unusual dish makes a lovely filling dinner. Make the tomato sauce first and reheat it when you are ready to cook the eggs.

Suitable for: Proteins and Healthy Fats, Better Carbs

Makes 2 portions • Ready in 50 minutes

1 tsp olive oil

1 shallot, peeled and finely chopped

1 red pepper, deseeded and finely chopped

1 garlic clove, peeled and finely chopped

1 courgette, peeled and finely chopped

1 tbsp tomato puree

½ tsp mild chilli powder

¼ tsp ground cinnamon

¼ tsp ground cumin

½ tsp salt

1 × 400g can chopped tomatoes

1 x 400g can chickpeas in water

small handful of flat-leaf parsley (10g), chopped

4 medium eggs at room temperature

- Heat the oil in a saucepan, add the shallot and red pepper and fry gently for 5 minutes. Then add the garlic and courgette and cook for another minute or two. Add the tomato puree, spices and salt and stir through.

- Add the chopped tomatoes and chickpeas (soaking liquor and all) and increase the heat to medium. With the lid off the pan, simmer the sauce for 30 minutes – make sure it is gently bubbling throughout and allow it to reduce in volume by about one-third.

- Remove from the heat and stir in the chopped parsley. Divide the sauce into two portions.
- Preheat the oven to 200C/180C fan.
- When you are ready to cook the eggs, bring one portion of the tomato sauce up to a gentle simmer and transfer to a small oven-proof dish.
- Crack two eggs on the side of the dish and lower them gently into the stew. Cover with foil and bake in the oven for 10-15 minutes. Serve the concoction in an individual bowl with the eggs floating on the top.

FRESH SAAG PANEER (V)

Using fresh spinach gives a whole new to this curry-house favourite. You can use pre-cooked rice for this dish, such as Tilda steamed rice, to make it easier.

Suitable for: Proteins and Healthy Fats

Makes 1 portion • Ready in 20 minutes

1 tsp olive oil
....
100g paneer, cut into cubes
....
Salt and freshly ground black pepper
....
1 shallot, chopped
....
1 small thumb (2cm) fresh ginger,
peeled and cut into matchsticks
....
1 clove garlic, peeled and thinly sliced
....
1 green chilli, deseeded and finely sliced
....
50g cherry tomatoes, halved
....
¼ tsp ground coriander
....
¼ tsp ground cumin
....
¼ tsp ground turmeric
....
½ tsp salt
....
50g fresh spinach leaves
....
Small handful fresh coriander,
chopped (optional)
....

- Heat the oil in a wide lidded frying pan over a high heat. Season the paneer generously with salt and pepper and toss into the pan. Fry for a few minutes until golden, stirring often. Remove from the pan with a slotted spoon and set aside.

- Reduce the heat and add the shallot. Fry for 5 minutes before adding the ginger, garlic and chilli.

Cook for another couple of minutes before adding the cherry tomatoes. Put the lid on the pan and cook for a further 5 minutes.

• Add the spices and salt, then stir. Return the paneer to the pan and stir until coated. Add the spinach and coriander to the pan and put the lid on. Allow the spinach to wilt for 1–2 minutes, then stir together thoroughly. Serve immediately.

CREAMY BAKED SALMON WITH MANGE TOUT

It's the fresh and herby dressing that makes this salmon dish really special.

Suitable for: Proteins and Healthy Fats

Serves 1 • Ready in 25 minutes

1 skinless salmon fillet, about 130g
....
salt and freshly ground black pepper
....
1 tsp olive oil
....
1 tsp mayonnaise
....
1 tbsp natural yogurt
....
1 tbsp rice wine
....
2 fresh mint leaves, finely chopped
....
2 spring onions, trimmed and sliced
....
100g mange tout, trimmed
....

- Preheat the oven to 200C/180C fan.

- Place the salmon fillet on a baking tray. Season with salt and pepper and rub the olive oil over the top. Bake in the oven for 16-18 minutes until just cooked through.

- In a small bowl, combine the mayonnaise, yogurt, rice wine, mint leaves and spring onions. Leave for 5-10 minutes for the flavours to develop.

- Boil or steam the mange tout according to the pack instructions.

- Arrange the warm mange tout on a plate. Lightly flake the salmon with a fork and arrange over the mange tout. Finally pour over the dressing. Serve immediately.

SPANISH BAKED PRAWNS

I love this easy prawn dish. You can use fresh or frozen prawns so it really is a no-brainer! It can be served with rice during the Better Carbs phase.

Suitable for: Proteins and Healthy Fats, Better Carbs

SERVES 2 • Ready in 15 minutes

2 tbsp extra-virgin olive oil
2 tbsp tomato purée
1 red chilli, seeded and finely chopped
2 cloves garlic, minced
1 tsp paprika
½ tsp dried dill or 1 tsp fresh
2 tbsp white wine vinegar
Few drops of Tabasco
200ml passata
250g cooked and peeled prawns (fresh or frozen)

- Preheat the oven to 230C/210C fan/450F/gas mark 8. In a small bowl or jug mix together the olive oil, tomato purée, chilli, garlic, paprika, dill, white wine vinegar, Tabasco and passata.

- Arrange the prawns in a small baking dish and pour the dressing over.

- Bake in the oven for 7 minutes for fresh prawns or 10 minutes for frozen.

GARLIC BUTTER CHICKEN

A very flavoursome chicken salad.

Suitable for: Proteins and Healthy Fats

Serves 2 • Ready in 15 minutes

2 cloves garlic, peeled and crushed

1 tbsp extra virgin olive oil

½ tsp dried oregano/mixed herbs

Freshly ground black pepper

20g butter, at room temperature

2 × 150g skinless chicken breast
fillets, cut into strips

80g rocket leaves

½ red onion, cut into very thin strips

Large handful (20g) parsley,
roughly chopped

½ cucumber, halved lengthways, deseeded

with a teaspoon and sliced

1 tsp white wine vinegar

- In a small bowl, combine the garlic, olive oil, dried herbs and black pepper. Set aside 1 teaspoon of the mixture to dress the salad. Add the butter to the bowl and mix until you have a smooth paste.

- Add the garlic butter to the chicken strips and use your hands to rub the butter all over the chicken pieces.

- Head a wide frying pan to a medium heat and when hot toss in the chicken strips. Cook for 10–14 minutes until browned and fully cooked, stirring regularly. Remove from the pan. The chicken can be used hot or cold in the salad.

- Arrange the rocket, red onion, parsley and cucumber over two serving plates. Add the white wine vinegar to the set aside garlic oil and pour over the two salads. Top with the cooked chicken.

SESAME CHICKEN SALAD

An unusual salad but very addictive.

Suitable for: Proteins and Healthy Fats

Serves 2 • Ready in 12 minutes

1 tbsp sesame seeds

1 cucumber, peeled, halved lengthways, deseeded with a teaspoon and sliced

100g baby kale, roughly chopped

60g pak choi, very finely shredded

½ red onion, very finely sliced

Large handful (20g) parsley, chopped

150g cooked chicken, shredded

For the dressing:

1 tbsp extra virgin olive oil

1 tsp sesame oil

Juice of 1 lime

1 tsp clear honey

2 tsp soy sauce

- Toast the sesame seeds in a dry frying pan for 2 minutes until lightly browned and fragrant. Transfer to a plate to cool.
- In a small bowl, mix together the olive oil, sesame oil, lime juice, honey and soy sauce to make the dressing.
- Place the cucumber, kale, pak choi, red onion and parsley in a large bowl and gently mix together. Pour over the dressing and mix again.
- Distribute the salad between two plates and top with the shredded chicken. Sprinkle over the sesame seeds just before serving.

ROAST CHICKEN AND PEANUTS

I think I might be addicted to the peanut dressing.

Suitable for: Proteins and Healthy Fats

Serves 2 • Ready in 15 minutes

60g small broccoli florets

150g cooked and cooled basmati rice

60g baby kale, chopped

60g young spinach leaves, chopped

Small handful (10g) parsley,
roughly chopped

200g cooked chicken breast, sliced

10g sesame seeds

For the dressing:

1 heaped tsp smooth peanut butter

10g creamed coconut dissolved
in 30ml boiling water

Juice of ½ lime

½ tsp brown sugar

½ tsp sesame oil

- Steam the broccoli over a pan of boiling water for 5 minutes or until just tender.

- Put the rice in a large bowl and break up any clumps with a fork. Add the kale, spinach, broccoli and parsley and stir gently.

- Add the dissolved coconut to the peanut butter a little bit at a time. Stir each time to ensure a smooth consistency. Add the lime juice, brown sugar and sesame oil. Divide the dressing in half and pour one half over the rice and greens and stir. Pour the rest of the dressing over the cooked chicken and stir gently until the chicken is fully coated.

- Scoop the dressed chicken over the greens and serve with the sesame seeds sprinkled over the top.

JAPANESE NOODLE SALAD

This salad is unusual, fresh and delicious.

Suitable for: Proteins and Healthy Fats

SERVES 4 • *Ready in 25 minutes*

2 cucumbers, washed
1 tbsp olive oil
200g minced beef
2 tsp Chinese five-spice powder
2 cloves garlic, finely grated
1 large thumb-sized piece of ginger, peeled and finely grated
250g cooked king prawns
2 heaped tsp brown sugar
6 spring onions, trimmed and finely sliced
Juice of 1 lime
1 tsp nam pla fish sauce
2 tsp tamari (Japanese wheat-free soy sauce)
1 red chilli, seeded and finely sliced
Handful of fresh coriander, chopped
2 fresh mint leaves, chopped
Freshly ground black pepper

- Use a vegetable peeler along the full length of the

cucumber, cut long flat noodles. Go down one side until you reach seeds, turn a quarter and start again. Repeat all round each cucumber. Spread out the cucumber over several sheets of kitchen paper and set aside.

- Heat the oil in a wide pan over a medium heat and add the minced beef and five-spice powder. Fry until well browned. Add the garlic, ginger, prawns, brown sugar and spring onions. Cook for 3–4 minutes.
- Place the cucumber noodles in a large bowl with the lime juice, nam pla, tamari, red chilli, coriander, mint and black pepper. Stir through and divide between four plates. Serve the beef and prawn mixture over the noodles. Serve hot or cold.

TIPS AND TRICKS: PROTEINS AND HEALTHY FATS

Breakfast

As I've mentioned before, eggs are your friend during the Proteins and Healthy Fats phase. If you like eggs for breakfast then go for it, especially if you're doing exercise later. I would recommend no more than 2 eggs (3 for a man) a day. So if you choose eggs for breakfast, try and avoid them for lunch or dinner.

Here's another quirky breakfast idea if you're really desperate: 2 babybel (or 40g of any other mild cheese such as gouda) with an apple. Wouldn't recommend for every day of this phase but in desperate times it's an option.

Lunch

A ready made salad with meat or cheese is a pretty good option. Practically any shop worth its salt will do a range of salads. M&S and Pret have a particularly good range. Choose a salad with chicken, fish, shellfish, red meat etc and no potatoes. You are allowed the dressing too, go for a vinaigrette style in preference.

Dinner

As always, if you only cook one meal for yourself a day then make it dinner. There is a huge range of options, many ready in 15 minutes or less. Or you could make a bigger portion meal such as the chicken cassoulet and have it ready for days when you get home late. If you really are absolutely stuck then go for a ready-made salad similar to the lunch options.

RECIPES: BETTER CARBS

Breakfast

Everyday oats

Bircher Muesli

Grilled Portobello Mushrooms

Raspberry Smoothie

Nutty Banana Energy Bars

Lunch

Mexican Chicken Soup

Mexican Bean Soup (V)

Falafel Lunchbox Salad (V)

Carrot and Coriander Soup

Puy Lentil and Feta Salad (V)

Spicy Sweet Potato Soup (V)

Tinned Salmon and Bean 'Salad'

Moroccan Chickpea Stew (V)

Hearty Ham Soup

Spicy Ramen with Rice Noodles (V)

Dinner

Mushroom and Blackbean Stir-fry (V)

Lightly Spiced Prawns with Vegetable Rice

Peanut Butter and Lime Prawns

Bean Burgers with New Potatoes and Mange Tout (V)

Vegetarian Curry Pot (V)

Warm Prawn and Avocado Salad

Parmesan Chicken

Mediterranean Lamb Hotpot

Lentil and Mushroom Bolognaise (V)

Sweet and Sour Chicken

Breakfast

EVERYDAY OATS

This is another oaty favourite of mine and can be
ready on the table in 2 minutes flat. Use your own Chia
Choc Granola for this recipe (it makes it go further!) or
use good quality shop-bought.

Suitable for: Detox and De-stress, Better Carbs

SERVES 1 • *Ready 2 mins*

30g jumbo oats

200ml milk

1 tbsp Greek yoghurt

10g granola

• Simply mix the oats, milk and yoghurt together in a
bowl, sprinkle the granola over the top and enjoy.

BIRCHER MUESLI

This is one of my favourite breakfast dishes at the moment. Make it up in a few minutes, tip it back into the yoghurt pot and it's ready to serve up for breakfast for the next few days. Be sure to use a yoghurt with no added sugars or flavourings and check that it is not low fat.

Suitable for: Detox and De-stress, Better Carbs

SERVES 4 • Ready in 2 mins

500g natural yoghurt

1 tbsp elderflower cordial

20g dried apricots, "Easy Microwave Porridge" on page 68chopped

50g jumbo rolled oats

- Simply tip the yoghurt out into a bowl and stir through the stevia, elderflower cordial, cranberries and oats. If it's too thick, add a little water and stir again.
- Serve immediately or scoop back into the yoghurt pot and chill overnight so the oats and yoghurt are soaked through and ready for tomorrow's breakfast.

GRILLED PORTOBELLO MUSHROOMS

Mushrooms are a much over-looked breakfast dish.

Suitable for: Better Carbs

Serves 1 • Ready in 15 minutes

2 flat open or portobello mushrooms
1 tsp extra-virgin olive oil
½ garlic clove, peeled and crushed
1 tsp chopped fresh parsley
1 medium tomato
salt and freshly ground black pepper

- Preheat the grill.
- Prepare the mushrooms by brushing off any soil and cutting out the stalks. Finely chop the stalks and mix in a small bowl with the olive oil, garlic and parsley.
- Cut the tomato in half, scoop out and discard all the seeds, then finely chop the tomato flesh and add to the bowl.
- Place the mushrooms open side down on a grill pan and grill for 4 minutes. Remove the mushrooms from the grill pan and turn them over. Distribute the garlic and tomato mixture evenly over the mushrooms, season with salt and pepper and grill for a further 6 minutes. Serve immediately.

RASPBERRY SMOOTHIE

If you don't have fresh raspberries, use defrosted frozen raspberries (or similar berries).

Suitable for: Better Carbs

Serves 1 • Ready in 2 minutes

approx 20 raspberries, washed
½ banana
2 tbsp greek yogurt
200ml semi-skimmed milk

• Place all the ingredients in a blender and whizz until smooth. Serve immediately.

NUTTY BANANA ENERGY BARS

Using quinoa as well as oats in these bars adds a slight nutty taste.

Suitable for: Detox and De-stress, Better Carbs

Makes 16 bars • Ready in 1 hour 15 minutes

1 tsp mild olive oil

50g quinoa, well rinsed

170g porridge oats

1 tsp ground cinnamon

1 tsp baking powder

1 tbsp desiccated coconut

pinch of salt

50g dried cranberries

30g pecans, chopped

3 medium very ripe bananas, mashed

1 large egg, beaten

50g maple syrup

1 tbsp mild olive oil oil

2 tsp vanilla extract

• Line a 25 × 25cm baking tray with two pieces of baking parchment, forming a cross shape so that all the sides are covered and rub the teaspoon of mild olive oil all over. Place the quinoa and 125ml water in a small saucepan and bring to the boil. Reduce the heat and simmer gently for 12–15 minutes or until the liquid is just absorbed. Remove from the heat and rest, covered, for 5 minutes. Transfer to a bowl and fluff with a fork. Leave to cool completely.

- Preheat the oven to 160C/140C fan/325F/Gas mark 3.
- Place the oats, cinnamon, baking powder, desiccated coconut and salt in a large bowl and mix thoroughly. Then mix in the dried cranberries and chopped pecans.
- Add the mashed bananas, beaten egg, maple syrup, oil and vanilla to the quinoa and stir until just combined. Add the banana mixture to the oat mixture and loosely mix.
- Press the batter into the prepared baking tray and bake in the oven for 35–40 minutes. Leave to cool completely in the tray.
- When cool, lift out using the baking parchment and transfer to a chopping board. Cut into 16 bars. Wrap individually in clingfilm and store in the refrigerator for up to a week.

Lunch

MEXICAN CHICKEN SOUP

This delicately spiced soup is warming and filling. Feel free to add a fresh chilli if you like it hot!

Suitable for: Proteins and Healthy Fats, Better Carbs

Makes 2 portions • Ready in 1 hour

2 chicken drumsticks

1 shallot, peeled and roughly chopped

1 small carrot, peeled and roughly chopped

1 stick celery, trimmed and finely chopped

500ml water

1x400g can chopped tomatoes

1 green pepper, deseeded and chopped

1 clove garlic, peeled and crushed

1 tsp dried mixed herbs

½ tsp paprika

½ tsp smoked paprika

¼ tsp turmeric

¼ tsp ground cumin

1 tsp salt

Freshly ground black pepper

1 tsp mild chilli powder

20g (handful) flat leaf parsley, stalks removed and chopped

• Place the chicken drumsticks, shallots, carrot and

celery in a large saucepan. Pour over the water and bring up to a simmer. Cook for 20 minutes, then remove the chicken drumsticks with a slotted spoon and set aside to cool.

- Add the chopped tomatoes, green pepper and garlic and bring back up to simmering point. Add the dried herbs, paprika, smoked paprika, turmeric, cumin, salt, black pepper and chilli powder, then simmer gently for 30 minutes.

- Remove the skin from the drumsticks and pull as much chicken as possible off the bone. Shred the chicken meat and return it to the pan. Remove from the heat and stir in the parsley.

MEXICAN BEAN SOUP (V)

An alternative to the Mexican chicken soup.

Suitable for: Better Carbs

Serves 2 • Ready in 50 minutes

1 tsp olive oil
1 shallot, peeled and roughly chopped
1 small carrot, peeled and roughly chopped
1 stick celery, trimmed and finely chopped
500ml water
1x400g can chopped tomatoes
1 green pepper, deseeded and chopped
1 clove garlic, peeled and crushed
1 tsp dried mixed herbs
½ tsp paprika
½ tsp smoked paprika
¼ tsp turmeric
¼ tsp ground cumin
1 tsp salt
Freshly ground black pepper
1 tsp mild chilli powder
½ x 400g can blackbeans
20g (handful) flat leaf parsley, stalks removed and chopped

- Heat the oil in a large saucepan. Add the shallot, carrot and celery and fry gently for about 5 minutes.
- Add the water, chopped tomatoes, green pepper and garlic and bring a gentle simmer. Add the dried herbs,

paprika, smoked paprika, turmeric, cumin, salt, black pepper and chilli powder, then cook gently for 30 minutes. Add the black beans, soaking liquor and all, and cook for a further 15 minutes.

• Stir through the parsley just before serving.

FALAFEL LUNCHBOX SALAD (V)

This may look like a lot of work but actually you are making 4 lunches here, plenty for the whole of one Better Carbs phase. Each part of the lunchbox – the falafel, tahini sauce and parsley salad – can be made in advance and will keep for several days in the fridge.

When you want to serve, just place the salad in a serving dish or container, add the falafel and drizzle on the tahini sauce. If it's a portable lunchbox you need, just store one portion of tahini sauce in a small lidded container and pour over just before eating.

Suitable for: Detox and De-stress, Better Carbs

Serves 4 • Ready in 45 minutes

For the falafel:

80g unsalted shelled pistachios

30g sesame seeds

¼ tsp ground cumin

¼ tsp ground coriander

¼ tsp ground turmeric

½ clove garlic, peeled and sliced 30g flat-leaf parsley

Salt and freshly ground black pepper For the tahini sauce:

2 tbsp (30g) tahini

1 tbsp white wine vinegar

Juice of ½ lemon

2 tbsp extra virgin olive oil

½ clove garlic, peeled

30g flat-leaf parsley, roughly chopped Pinch of salt

For the parsley salad:

150g couscous

Juice of 2 lemons

1 tbsp extra virgin olive oil

Salt and freshly ground black pepper

¼ tsp ground cinnamon

¼ tsp ground coriander

Pinch of ground cloves

Pinch of ground ginger

4 tomatoes, finely chopped

2 spring onions, finely sliced

50g flat-leaf parsley, stalks discarded,
leaves very finely chopped

- To make the falafel balls, simply pulse all the ingredients in a food processor until you have coarse breadcrumbs. Remove heaped teaspoons from the food processor and form into balls by rolling in your hands. Set aside or refrigerate in a lidded container until needed.

- To make the tahini sauce, place all the ingredients in a blender and blend until smooth. Add a little water to thin if necessary. Set aside or refrigerate in a lidded container until needed.

- To make the parsley salad, place the couscous in a bowl and add the lemon juice, extra virgin olive oil and plenty of salt and pepper. Add all the spices, erring on the side of caution especially with the cinnamon and cloves. Stir to combine. Pour over enough water so that the couscous is generously covered. Leave to rest for approximately 10 minutes until all the water is absorbed and the couscous has swelled and is cooked 'al dente'. Keep topping up the water when required during the rest period. Meanwhile combine the tomato, spring onion and parsley. Mix the salad into the spicy couscous and allow the flavours to meld for at least 5 minutes before serving.

CARROT AND CORIANDER SOUP

This classic soup is a breeze to make and is very warming.

Suitable for: Better Carbs

Serves 4 • Ready in 30 minutes

1 large onion, peeled and chopped
500g carrots, about 6 medium
1 small potato (100g), peeled and chopped
1 tsp ground coriander
1 litre vegetable stock (fresh or made with 2 cubes)
large handful of fresh coriander
freshly ground black pepper
4 tsp extra virgin olive oil

- Simply place the onion, carrots, potato and ground coriander in a large saucepan and pour in the stock. Bring to the boil, reduce the heat and simmer for 15-18 minutes until tender.

- Blitz in a blender or food processor with the fresh coriander until smooth. Return the soup to the pan and reheat gently.

- Serve with lashings of black pepper and a drizzle (1 teaspoon) of extra virgin olive oil.

PUY LENTIL AND FETA SALAD (V)

This is an easy salad that you can put together using mainly ingredients from the store cupboard.

Suitable for: Better Carbs

SERVES 2 • Ready in 10 minutes

1 tbsp balsamic vinegar

1 tsp walnut oil

2 tsp extra-virgin olive oil

½ tsp English mustard

Salt and freshly ground pepper

1 x 400g tin ready-to-eat
puy lentils, drained

30g roasted red peppers from a
tin or jar, drained and chopped

30g rocket leaves

6 cherry tomatoes, halved

60g feta cheese, cut into rough cubes

30g walnuts, halved

• Prepare the dressing by mixing together the balsamic vinegar, walnut oil, olive oil, English mustard and salt and pepper. In a large bowl combine the lentils with the roasted red peppers, rocket leaves and cherry tomatoes. Stir about three-quarters of the dressing through. Arrange the feta and walnuts over the top and finally drizzle over the rest of the dressing.

SPICY SWEET POTATO SOUP (V)

This is a very quick and easy soup.

Suitable for: Detox and De-stress, Better Carbs

Serves 2 • Ready in 30 minutes

1 tsp olive oil
....
2 sweet potatoes, peeled
and roughly chopped
....
2 garlic cloves, peeled and crushed
....
1 tsp medium curry powder
....
½ tsp smoked paprika
....
1 tsp cornflour
....
½ vegetable stock cube
....
1 tsp tomato ketchup
....
juice of 1 lemon
....

- Heat the oil in a saucepan, add the sweet potatoes and garlic and fry for 4–5 minutes. Sprinkle in the curry powder, paprika and cornflour and stir-fry for 1 more minute.

- Add 2 tablespoons water and stir to form a paste (this is to stop the cornflour going lumpy) before adding approximately 500-700ml water (you can always add more later). Crumble in the stock cube and add the ketchup and lemon juice. Bring to the boil, then reduce the heat and simmer for 15–20 minutes or until the sweet potato is tender.

- Transfer to a blender and blend until smooth, then serve.

TINNED SALMON AND BEAN 'SALAD'

This is a fantastic 'store cupboard' salad. Although it serves two, I tend to make it just for me and refrigerate half. It keeps well in the fridge for up to two days and I think tastes even better the next day!

Suitable for: Proteins and Healthy Fats, Better Carbs

Serves 2 • Ready in 15 minutes

100g green beans, fresh or frozen

½ red onion, peeled and cut into half rings

1 tbsp extra virgin olive oil

juice of 1 lemon

1 × 200g can salmon

1 × 400g can mixed beans,
rinsed and drained

salt and freshly ground black pepper

- Heat a small pan of water until boiling. Add the green beans and simmer for 3–4 minutes (fresh) or 5–6 minutes (frozen). Drain and leave to cool.

- Place the sliced onion in a small microwaveable bowl. Add the olive oil and lemon juice. Cover the bowl with clingfilm and microwave on high for 2 minutes. Leave to rest, covered, for a further 2 minutes.

- In a larger bowl, mix together the salmon, mixed beans and green beans. Pour the softened onion, oil and lemon juice over and combine. Season with salt and pepper. This can be served immediately or refrigerated in individual portions.

MOROCCAN CHICKPEA STEW (V)

This unusual and earthy Moroccan stew is a warming winter dish which works equally well as a main meal or as a 'tupperware lunch'.

Suitable for: Detox and De-stress, Better Carbs

Serves 4 • Ready in 1 hour

1 tbsp olive oil

1 onion, chopped

1 clove garlic, finely chopped

1 red pepper, seeded and diced

1 aubergine, cut into chunks

2 tsp ground cumin

½ tsp ground cinnamon

2 tsp ground coriander

1 tbsp tomato purée

2 tbsp harissa paste

1 x 400g tin chickpeas, rinsed and drained

150g red lentils

20g fresh flat-leaf parsley

2 tomatoes, roughly chopped

Juice of 1 lemon

Salt and freshly ground black pepper

• Heat the oil in a large pan, add the onion and fry for 7–8 minutes until translucent. Add the garlic, pepper and aubergine and fry for another 5 minutes. Add in the spices, tomato purée and harissa paste and stir through for a minute or two. Add the chickpeas and lentils and cover generously with 800– 900ml of just boiled water. Bring to the boil and simmer vigorously for 10 minutes. Then reduce the heat and simmer gently for a further 15 minutes. Keep topping up the water if it threatens to dry out.

- Remove from the heat and stir in the parsley, tomatoes and lemon juice. Season with salt and pepper and serve immediately.

HEARTY HAM SOUP

With lentils and pearl barley this soup is REALLY filling.

Suitable for: Detox and De-stress, Better Carbs

Serves 4 • Ready in 1 hour 30 minutes

1 tbsp olive oil
1 onion, finely diced
2 carrots, diced
30g red lentils
30g green puy lentils
30g pearl barley
750ml chicken stock, fresh or made with 1½ stock cubes
250g cooked ham or gammon, cut into bite sized pieces
1 medium potato, peeled and diced

- Heat the oil in a large saucepan or casserole and fry the onions and carrots very gently for 10 minutes until the onions are transparent.

- Rinse the lentils and pearl barley, stir into the pan and then add the stock. Bring to the boil, cover and simmer for 45 minutes. Add the ham and potato and simmer for a further 30 minutes.

SPICY RAMEN WITH RICE NOODLES (V)

This soup is incredibly satisfying and warming and can be made in under 10 minutes.

Suitable for: Detox and De-stress, Better Carbs

Serves 2 • Ready in 10 minutes

50g (2 heaped tablespoons) Miso paste
2 tsp mirin
2 tbsp dark soy sauce
1 inch fresh ginger, peeled and grated
100g spring greens or savoy cabbage, thinly sliced
1 carrot, peeled and cut into very fine batons
100g Shiitake mushrooms, washed and sliced
100g beansprouts
200g fresh rice noodles

- Bring 800ml water to boiling point in a saucepan. Stir in the miso paste, mirin, soy and ginger. Stir until the miso is dissolved. Add in the greens, carrot and mushrooms. Put the lid on the pan and simmer gently for 5 minutes.

- Add the beansprouts and rice noodles to the ramen. Cook for a further 2 minutes before serving.

Dinner

MUSHROOM AND BLACKBEAN STIR-FRY (V)

This stir-fry is delicious and filling.

Suitable for: Detox and De-stress, Better Carbs

Serves 1 • Ready in 20 minutes

1 tsp water
....
1 tsp rice wine
....
1 tsp tomato puree
....
½ tsp brown sugar
....
1 tbsp light soy sauce
....
½ clove garlic, peeled and grated
....
½ thumb (2cm) fresh ginger,
peeled and grated
....
1 tsp olive oil
....
½ tsp walnut oil
....
50g shiitake mushrooms, sliced
....
100g chestnut mushrooms,
washed and sliced
....
2 spring onions, trimmed and shredded
....
100g pak choi, cut into thin slices
....
30g beansprouts
....
½ x 400g can blackbeans,
rinsed and drained
....

- In a small bowl, mix the water, rice wine, tomato puree, brown sugar and soy sauce. Add the garlic and ginger and stir together.

- In a wok or large frying pan, heat the olive and walnut oils together on a high heat. Add both types of mushrooms to the pan and stir-fry for 2-3 minutes until cooked and glossy. Then add the spring onions, pak choi and beansprouts and stir-fry until the pak choi has wilted.

- Reduce the heat to low, then stir in the blackbeans and add the sauce. Allow the sauce to bubble for a minute then remove from the heat and serve immediately.

LIGHTLY SPICED PRAWNS WITH VEGETABLE RICE

Although this has quite a few ingredients, the majority should be cupboard staples. If you don't like prawns feel free to substitute with chicken (which you should add with the shallot rather than at the end). Note also that you can use a packet of pre-cooked rice for this dish to make it even easier. I use Tilda brown basmati steamed rice.

Suitable for: Better Carbs

Serves 1 • Ready in 20 minutes

1 tsp olive oil

1 clove

1 bay leaf

1 shallot, chopped

½ red pepper, deseeded and chopped

1 clove garlic, peeled and thinly sliced

1 red or green chilli, deseeded
and sliced (optional)

½ tsp mild chilli powder

½ tsp paprika

¼ tsp ground turmeric

¼ tsp ground cumin

¼ tsp cinnamon

½ tsp salt

1 fresh tomato, roughly chopped

30g frozen soya/edamame beans

1 tbsp water

125g raw king prawns (if frozen,
cook for a little longer/defrost

as per pack instructions)
....
100g cooked and cooled basmati rice
....
20g young leaf spinach, stalks removed
....
Small handful fresh coriander,
chopped (optional)
....

- In a wide lidded frying pan, heat the oil on a medium heat. Add the cloves and bay leaf. Add the onion and red pepper. Stir, turn the heat to low and place the lid on the pan. Cook for 5 minutes.

- Remove the lid from the pan. Add the garlic, chilli, chilli powder, paprika, turmeric, ground cumin, cinnamon and salt and fry for a further minute. Add the chopped tomatoes, soya beans and water. Replace the lid on the pan and cook gently for 7 minutes.

- Take the lid off the pan and remove the cloves and bay leaf. Add the prawns and cook until just pink. Then add the rice, stir thoroughly and warm through. Finally, stir through the spinach and coriander just before serving.

PEANUT BUTTER AND LIME PRAWNS

You make this amazing marinade for the prawns and then use it as a dipping sauce. Trust me – it's amazing!

Suitable for: Better Carbs

Serves 1 • Ready in 20 minutes

For the marinade:
....
Juice of ½ lime
....
1 tsp (10g) peanut butter
....
1 tbsp water
....
½ tsp tomato puree
....
½ clove garlic, crushed
....
¼ tsp ground ginger
....
125g raw king prawns
....
For the rice:
....
100g cooked and cooled basmati rice
....
2 tomatoes, chopped
....
5cm cucumber, cut into small cubes
....
1 spring onion, finely chopped
....
Juice of ½ lime
....
Salt and pepper
....

- Combine all the marinade ingredients in a wide bowl and stir together thoroughly. Add the king prawns and leave to marinate for 15-20 minutes.

- Place the cooked rice in a bowl and mush gently with a fork to remove any lumps. Add the tomatoes, cucumber and spring onion. Squeeze over the lime juice and season with salt and pepper. Stir well and leave for the flavours to develop.

- Remove the prawns from the marinade and shake off into the bowl so you don't lose any precious marinade. Place on kitchen paper to dry. Heat a frying pan on a medium heat and add the marinade. Heat gently and allow to bubble for 2 minutes, adding a little more water if necessary, before transferring to a small bowl for dipping.

- Turn the heat up to high and add the prawns. Fry for 3-4 minutes, stirring regularly until cooked through.

- To serve, place the rice on a plate and arrange the prawns over the top. Serve with the dipping sauce on the side.

BEAN BURGERS WITH NEW POTATOES AND MANGE TOUT (V)

Delicious and really quick to prepare.

Suitable for: Detox and De-stress, Better Carbs

Serves 1 • Ready in 20 minutes

120g, about 3 medium, new potatoes
....
½ × 400g tin cannellini beans,
rinsed and drained
....
1 tsp tomato purée
....
1 tsp cornflour
....
1 spring onion, trimmed and chopped
....
½ clove garlic, peeled and crushed
....
½ tsp mild chilli powder
....
¼ tsp ground turmeric
....
Salt and freshly ground black pepper
....
1 tsp mayonnaise
....
1 tbsp natural yogurt
....
1 tsp rice wine
....
2 fresh mint leaves, finely chopped
....
2 spring onions, trimmed and sliced
....
100g mange tout, trimmed
....
1 tsp olive oil
....

- Quarter the potatoes and steam or boil until tender. Add the mange tout for the last 4-5 minutes of cooking time. Drain and cover.

- Place the beans in a large bowl and use a potato masher or fork to thoroughly mash the beans. Add the tomato purée, cornflour, spring onion, garlic, chilli powder and turmeric. Season generously with salt and pepper. Mix well.

- Divide the mixture into two portions and form into balls, then flatten a little to form a burger. If you have time, chill for 20 minutes or keep refrigerated until needed. The burgers will hold their shape slightly better if chilled but will be just as delicious if cooked straight away.

- In a small bowl, combine the mayonnaise, yogurt, rice wine, mint leaves and spring onions. Leave for 5-10 minutes for the flavours to develop.

- Heat the oil in a frying pan over a medium heat. Add the burgers to the pan and cook for 3–4 minutes on one side. Turn with a fish slice and flatten a little more if necessary. Cook for a further 3–4 minutes until golden brown.

- Arrange the warm potatoes and mange tout over a plate. Place the burgers on the top. Finally pour over the dressing. Serve immediately.

VEGETARIAN CURRY POT (V)

I make this warming and filling curry pot an awful lot – it's a whole meal in a bowl. It re-heats beautifully from chilled or frozen and is definitely one of those dishes you'll want to keep stacked in your freezer for a rainy day.

Suitable for: Detox and De-stress, Better Carbs

SERVES 4 • Ready in 1 hour

1 tbsp rapeseed oil

1 onion, finely chopped

4 cloves garlic, finely sliced

1 large thumb-sized piece of ginger, peeled and cut into matchsticks

1 large chilli, seeded and cut into rings

1 red pepper, seeded and chopped

½ tsp turmeric

½ tsp cayenne pepper

1 tsp paprika

1 tsp mild chilli powder

1 tsp salt

250g puy lentils

1½ litres water, just boiled

200g peas, fresh or frozen

200g paneer, cut into cubes

2 tomatoes, roughly chopped

Juice of 1 lime

- Heat the oil in a large heavy-based pan over a low heat. Add the onion, garlic, ginger, chilli and red pepper. Cook slowly for about 10 minutes until soft. Stir through the spices and salt. Next add the puy lentils and give the mixture a really good stir. Add enough water to generously cover the lentils and bring up to a vigorous simmer. Cook on a high simmer for 10 minutes, adding more water when necessary.

• Reduce the heat to very low and continue to cook for a further 20 minutes. Add more water when needed. Stir frequently to prevent it sticking to the bottom of the pan. Add the peas, paneer and tomatoes. Cook for a further 10 minutes or until the peas are tender. Remove from the heat and stir in the lime juice. Adjust the seasoning if necessary.

WARM PRAWN AND AVOCADO SALAD

Puy lentils add a complex earthiness to this dish. They contain the best kind of carbohydrates plus protein and fibre. Best of all, they can be bought pre-cooked and are ready to eat in a jiffy.

Suitable for: Detox and De-stress, Better Carbs

SERVES 2 • Ready in 10 minutes

200g cooked king prawns
1 red chilli, seeded and finely chopped
Zest and juice of 1 lime
1 tbsp light soy sauce
1 tsp clear honey
½ x 400-g tin puy lentils, drained
1 avocado, peeled, stoned and sliced
4 radishes, washed, trimmed and finely sliced
Handful of fresh coriander, finely chopped (optional)
1 tsp sesame oil
2 pak choi, separated into leaves and ends removed

- Place the prawns in a bowl with the chilli, lime zest and half the lime juice. Mix together and set aside while you prepare the rest of the dish.
- In a small bowl, mix together the soy sauce, honey and the rest of the lime juice. Put the lentils, avocado, radishes and coriander, if using, in a large bowl and stir through the soy dressing. Heat the sesame oil

in a frying pan and toss in the pak choi. Fry over a high heat until just wilted. Add the prawns and their marinade and warm through for 1–2 minutes. Divide the lentil salad between two plates and put the prawns and pak choi on top. Serve immediately.

PARMESAN CHICKEN

This is a deliciously easy way to cook chicken, and it's great for both kids and adults. I like to serve it with new potatoes and peas.

Suitable for: Better Carbs

SERVES 2 • Ready in 15 minutes

2 tbsp plain flour

1 egg, lightly beaten

30g Parmesan, finely grated

2 chicken breasts, each cut into 4–5 strips

1–2 tbsp olive oil

Salt and freshly ground black pepper

- Place the flour, egg and Parmesan in three separate shallow bowls, adding salt and pepper to the Parmesan bowl. Prepare the chicken by dipping each piece first in the flour, then the egg and finally the Parmesan.

- Heat the oil in a large frying pan over a medium heat. Place the chicken strips in the pan, leaving as much space as possible between the pieces. Cook for 3–5 minutes each side until brown, crunchy and cooked through. Serve immediately.

MEDITERRANEAN LAMB HOTPOT

This simple dish is very flavoursome and makes a great one pot meal.

Suitable for: Better Carbs

SERVES 4 • Ready in 2 hours

1 large onion, chopped
600g diced lamb
600g fresh tomatoes, roughly chopped
400g new potatoes, halved
Zest and juice of ½ orange
2 tsp cumin seeds
200ml chicken stock, warmed
1 tbsp tomato purée
Pinch of sugar
2 bay leaves
Salt and freshly ground black pepper

- Preheat the oven to 210C/190C fan/400F/gas mark 6. Arrange the onion over the base of a deep baking dish. Add the lamb, tomatoes and new potatoes. Sprinkle over the orange zest and juice.

- Crush the cumin seeds lightly in a pestle and mortar and sprinkle over the lamb. Dissolve the tomato purée and sugar in the chicken stock and pour over the lamb. Tuck in the bay leaves and season generously with salt and pepper. Cover with foil and bake in the oven for 1½ hours, or until the meat is very tender.

LENTIL AND MUSHROOM BOLOGNAISE (V)

This bolognaise is so filling and versatile that you simply don't need the meat. There is enough here to serve six so you can freeze individual portions.

Suitable for: Detox and De-stress, Better Carbs

SERVES 6 • Ready in 1 hour 30 minutes

2 tbsp olive oil
1 large onion, chopped
250g mushrooms, washed and sliced
4 cloves garlic, sliced
1 carrot, peeled and chopped
1 green pepper, seeded and chopped
250g brown or green lentils
1 x 400g tin chopped tomatoes
1 bay leaf
500ml vegetable stock, fresh or made with 1 stock cube
½ tsp chilli flakes
200ml red wine

- In a large pan, heat the oil over a medium heat. Fry the onion for 5 minutes. Add the mushrooms, garlic, carrot and green pepper. Cook for 15–20 minutes until soft, stirring frequently. Stir in the lentils, then add the chopped tomatoes, bay leaf, vegetable stock and chilli flakes. Bring to the boil and cook on a vigorous heat for 10 minutes. Reduce the heat to medium/low, add the wine and cook for a further 20–30 minutes until the sauce is rich and thick.

SWEET AND SOUR CHICKEN

An easy, everyday supper. Serve with rice.

Suitable for: Better Carbs

SERVES 2 • *Ready in 15 minutes*

2 skinless chicken breasts, cut into strips
....
1 small onion, sliced
....
1 red pepper, seeded and sliced
....
½ head broccoli, cut into small florets
....
1 clove garlic, finely sliced
....
2 tsp cornflour
....
1 tbsp olive oil
....
1 tsp clear honey
....
1 tbsp white wine vinegar
....
1 tsp tomato purée
....
1 tsp soy sauce
....
½ tsp English mustard
....
50ml water
....
1 tbsp sherry
....

- Place the chicken, onion, pepper, broccoli and garlic in a bowl. Sprinkle over the cornflour and season with salt and pepper. Mix together thoroughly.

- Heat the oil in a wide pan over a medium heat. Toss in the chicken and vegetable mixture and cook, stirring every minute, until just cooked (about 8-10 minutes, depending on size).

- Meanwhile mix the honey, vinegar, tomato purée, soy sauce, English mustard, water & sherry in a small bowl. When the chicken is just cooked, stir in the sauce and allow to bubble gently for 2 minutes.

Lose a Stone in January

TIPS AND TRICKS: BETTER CARBS

Breakfast

A very healthy oat cereal with no added sugar. Also rolled oats are better than the smaller oat flakes. Try to avoid anything with low fat or fat free yogurt or milk. If you can manage it, go for porridge, it only takes a few minutes to make and is the only way to guarantee no added sugar.

Lunch

A fresh vegetable or bean soup is perfectly suitable. Look for good quality or freshly-made soup with recognisable ingredients. The orange vegetables (carrot, butternut, sweet potato) make particularly good soups for this phase.

You could also go for a shop-bought salad if you need to. During the Better Carbs phase you should get a salad with some carbs (normally rice, new potatoes or beans). Avoid red or processed meats in your salad, but chicken, cheese or fish are all fine.

Dinner

Please please go for a recipe that you cook yourself. There are many to choose from for this phase. If you're totally unprepared then a jacket potato with a little butter, half a can of reduced sugar beans (we like Heinz as they don't have added artificial sweeteners) and a smattering (20g max) of grated cheddar.

Here's how I cook a jacket potato in less than 15 minutes:

Pre-heat the oven to 220C/200C fan.

Wash the potato and dry with kitchen paper. Use the sharp end of a peeler to pull out any eyes or brown bits. Pierce all over with a fork, making sure you push the fork all the way in each time (this helps it cook evenly).

Microwave for 2 minutes on one side – 3 minutes if it's exceptionally large. Turn it over and microwave for 2 minutes more. If you are cooking more than one potato you should increase the time.

Transfer to the pre-heated oven and bake for 10 minutes.

Don't forget that during the Better Carbs phase you are allowed *fruit* and *dark chocolate*.

For the fruit, one portion with every meal is perfect. I wouldn't recommend banana except as a main breakfast option but all berries, cherries, citrus fruits like orange or satsuma, apples, pears, kiwis are all good. It is preferable to only have the fruit with or after a meal. You should find that by the time you reach a better carb phase, your blood sugar highs and lows are reduced so there'll be no need to reach for emergency fruit as a snack.

Dark chocolate (70%) is allowed as a replacement for the fruit after lunch or dinner. A 20g portion (normally six squares) is the maximum per day.

Win a NUTRiBULLET

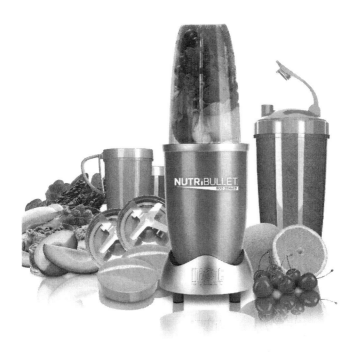

Fancy owning a super NutriBullet Pro 900?

Nutribullet Pro 900 unlocks the hidden nutrition inside super foods that are integral to our health.

I'm running a contest where you can win a NutriBullet. Here is the link where you can enter for free:

www.52recipes.co.uk/giveaways/nutribullet

20770056R00099

Printed in Great Britain
by Amazon